TAKE IT TO HEART

Your Complete Guide to
PREVENTING and TREATING
Heart Disease

ROB MYERS is board certified in both Internal Medicine and Cardiology in Canada and the United States and is a fellow of the Royal College of Physicians and Surgeons of Canada and the American College of Cardiology. Dr. Myers is currently a cardiologist at the coronary care unit at Sunnybrook Health Science Centre, the largest academic hospital in Canada. He lives in Toronto with his wife and two children.

TAKE IT TO HEART

Your Complete Guide to PREVENTING and TREATING Heart Disease

DR. ROB MYERS,

CARDIOLOGIST

ECW PRESS

The publication of *Take It to Heart* has been generously
supported by The Canada Council, the Ontario Arts Council,
and the Government of Canada through the Book
Publishing Industry Development Program.

CANADIAN CATALOGUING IN PUBLICATION DATA
Myers, Rob
Take it to heart : your complete guide
to preventing and treating heart disease
ISBN 1-55022-339-9
1. Heart
1. Title.
KE7709.G73 1996   342.714´0872   c96-990056-2

Illustrations by Domenic Pirone.

Imaging by ECW Type & Art, Oakville, Ontario.
Printed and bound by AGMV Marquis
Imprimeur, Cap-Saint-Ignace, Québec.

Distributed in Canada by General Distribution Services,
30 Lesmill Road, Don Mills, Ontario M3B 2T6.

Distributed in the United States by LPC Group,
1436 West Randolph Street, Chicago, Illinois, U.S.A. 60607.

Published by ECW PRESS,
2120 Queen Street East, Suite 200,
Toronto, Ontario M4E 1E2.

www.ecw.ca/press

PRINTED AND BOUND IN CANADA

Table of Contents

FOREWORD

Heart disease is the most common cause of death in North America. Despite this fact, few people understand what heart disease is and how to prevent it. Though many are familiar with catchwords like "heart attack," "cholesterol," or "coronary artery," they often lack a detailed understanding of these terms. This deficit may be acceptable when dealing with your car or the plumbing in your home, but when it comes to the health of you and your loved ones, basic knowledge about your heart may save your life.

This book will teach you about your cardiac risk factors and how to modify them to prevent a heart attack. The prescription, as you will discover, is quite simple. I shall provide you with accurate information upon which to base intelligent decisions. My goal is to dispel the fear of illness by making the subject of heart disease easier to understand. I want you to realize you can take control of much of your health, and I will tell you how to grab the reins. I hope you will also find this book entertaining.

I

INTRODUCTION

Health is similar to gambling since both revolve around improving one's odds. There is no 100% assurance that you will live longer by following my advice. There are no easy-to-pay installments of $19.95 and this book does not come with the world's smallest juicer. What I promise is scientific knowledge in a format that does not require a medical degree to understand. I guarantee that by following the healthier lifestyle described in these pages, you will sharply reduce your odds of developing heart disease. Not negate them, but reduce them.

As a cardiologist, I have noticed that most people with heart problems do not understand the risks. Though some prefer ignorance, the overwhelming majority are genuinely interested in learning more about their health. That interest may stem from their own brush with heart disease or perhaps illness in a friend or family member. Fear is classically a powerful motivator. As the proverb says, health is like a crown noticed only by the sick.

Some view medical information as plodding and mundane, but it does not have to be either. This book summarizes decades of research by thousands of scientists involving millions of patients. Utilizing the information on these pages, you will be able to modify your risk factors for heart disease and improve your chances of living longer and healthier. This material is not new. I have simply made it readily accessible in an easy-to-understand format.

If you have the motivation to improve your health and live longer, you are gazing at the tool to facilitate this change with surprisingly little effort. Those unwilling to modify their lifestyle by exercising, eating intelligently, and keeping that cigarette unlit will quickly discover that this book will make a better gift for someone else.

Morbidity & Mortality

Diseases in medicine are spoken of in terms of **morbidity** and **mortality**. Mortality is simply defined as death. Morbidity refers to the incapacitation that results from an illness. Although it is clear that heart disease kills, people may be less aware that heart disease causes morbidity. Many people with heart problems are robbed of their normal ability to function. They may be housebound, bedridden, or chronically hospitalized. They may find their activity levels so curtailed that showering becomes a marathon of breathlessness. Patients often sink into depression as they spend their golden years chained to a post of symptoms and hospital visits. Though modern medicine may provide a cure, doctors can often only ease the slope of a patient's demise.

I believe that a great deal of the death and suffering associated with cardiac disease is preventable. "Believe" is a misleading word, as I *know* this to be true based on clear scientific evidence. The major impediment to altering cardiac risk factors is a lack of **information**. A simple program of risk factor modification in easy-to-understand terminology is one of the most successful ways to live longer and healthier.

Many people die before exercising their education options. I have seen a middle-aged lawyer with a history of high blood pressure who was found slumped over his desk. I have treated a wife and mother whose cholesterol was "a little high" as her heart failed, badly damaged from a sudden heart attack. I have led many unsuccessful resuscitations of men and women on the threshold of their retirement years. Unfortunately, people in their 40s and 50s are not immune to this scourge. Many of these situations could have been prevented if the patients had altered their lifestyles.

Responsibility

Personal responsibility is the only way to successfully direct the course of your health. Reading these pages is an important first step in transforming your risks and implies a level of interest and motivation. I harbour no fantasies of converting the world to a life of soybean and treadmills. That doesn't even sound attractive to me. My goal is to inspire you to address your risk factors and improve your health.

I will provide you with information on the perils of smoking, which could start you on the road to quitting. What you decide to do after reading the chapter, however, is up to you. The same applies to improved eating habits. If you choose to continue to smoke a pack a day or gorge on fat-laden, vegetable-bereft meals, that is your choice. You have to police your own habits. Once you have the facts, the decision to continue practising high-risk behaviour becomes an educated one, and I believe in informed choices.

Unfortunately, many physicians do not have time for patient education. With the system of health care remuneration in North America, quantity (i.e., the number of patients seen by a doctor) is more cost-effective than the delivery of more complete quality care. This is not meant to imply that patients are not receiving quality care from their physicians. My point is that health care may occasionally be incomplete. If a doctor sees 10 patients a day and spends an hour reviewing risk factors, he or she probably won't be able to pay the bills. In place of this approach, a doctor schedules 20 patients in the same time frame, and a pill for blood pressure or cholesterol substitutes for education. As a result, patients must take the responsibility of educating themselves. This book is the beginning of that journey.

Language

Part of the difficulty in understanding medical concepts is the baffling array of perplexing terminology. Doctors learn thousands of medical terms over years of training. There is often insufficient emphasis on effective communication with patients. We essentially speak a foreign language to one another in our day-to-day business. Unfortunately, we tend to use the same language with patients. This is confusing and frustrating for patients, and it may leave them feeling alienated and intimidated. When a patient tells me their previous doctor didn't explain anything, what they are often saying is they didn't understand any of it. The following statement describes a heart attack: *The culprit lesion was the LAD with thrombotic occlusion and transmural infarction resulting in a dyskinetic apex.* In other words, the heart was damaged when its blood supply was blocked. Two very different ways to explain exactly the same problem. A patient who does not speak the same language as the doctor is one example where even special efforts may be unrewarding. In most cases, however, it takes very little effort to explain a medical problem in simple, easy-to-understand terms. This philosophy forms the vertebral column (backbone) of this book.

Anecdotes

Medical anecdotes are individual claims of success (or failure). They represent one person's story. "I drank spring water for a year and my arthritis is cured." If 1,000 people with arthritis drank spring water and 200 were cured of their arthritis, does that make it a miracle cure? What if I told you that another 1,000 people who drank what they thought was spring water, but was actually tap water, also had a cure rate of 20% (200 out of 1000)? This would be a study, which in this case proves that the extract is just as likely to cure arthritis as tap water (though you could guess which costs more). Therefore, anecdotes can never be extrapolated to apply to an entire population, unless they are part of a study.

I find no comfort in anecdotes, because by themselves, they have no scientific basis. A typical narrative, however, will gush with enthusiasm over a dramatic recovery from near death, using nothing but coffee enemas, candle wax, and the rib of a rhinoceros (which, incidentally, is high in cholesterol). Those who advocate alfalfa juice for medicinal benefit are usually selling it.

I do not advocate a homeopathic approach. It is difficult to compete with baseless claims which use unproven herbal remedies or elaborate schemes involving useless procedures. Colonic irrigation has never been shown to successfully combat heart disease. If inserting "natural and organic" compounds into every orifice truly reduced the chances of falling ill, then I would gladly partake. (Maybe not gladly, but I would do it anyway.)

Non-traditional approaches are often based on fear of what is not understood, and I sympathize with this. The world of medicine is very foreign to most people, which naturally leads to feelings of insecurity and intimidation. However, the solution lies in knowledge, not mysticism. The control sought by patients who turn to non-traditional approaches can be achieved with correct information. Remove the unknown, at least that part based on misunderstanding, and the fear will be eliminated with it.

I am a strong proponent of patients taking control of their health. Doctors need to be questioned, patients need to be educated, and diseases need to be understood. I simply have little patience for medical stories from the *National*

Enquirer or quasi-medical advice from people with unclear motives.

As patients age, health becomes a greater focus of time and worry, but with cardiac education it is never too late to learn. Whether your goal is to prevent the development of heart disease or to halt and even reverse its effects, the first step is to understand it. I can start you on that road. Scientific background is not necessary to understand how to lower your risk. In the following pages you will discover the education part of "education and modification of risk factors." You will learn everything from the effects of alcohol on heart disease to which foods contain hidden fats. Whether your interest is the safety of exercise, the effects of menopause, or the beauty (yes, beauty) of a high-fibre diet, read on, reduce your risk, and live longer.

POINTS TO REMEMBER

- **Educating yourself about your risk factors for heart disease will favourably change those risks.**

- **Heart disease can kill (mortality) and significantly decrease a person's functional capacity (morbidity).**

- **Learning about your health can be easy if the terminology is simplified.**

- **Learn about your health by questioning your doctor. If your doctor has no time to answer your questions, find one who does.**

- **Beware of simple remedies sold by those who stand to make a profit. If it isn't proven, it may not be true, it may not help you, and it may harm you.**

2

RISK FACTORS
& HEART DISEASE

There are a number of cardiac risk factors which dramatically increase the chances of developing heart disease. The more risks a person has, the more dramatic this increase will be (figure 1). As shown in table 1, risk factors are divided into those that can be modified and those that cannot. This chapter provides information on some of those

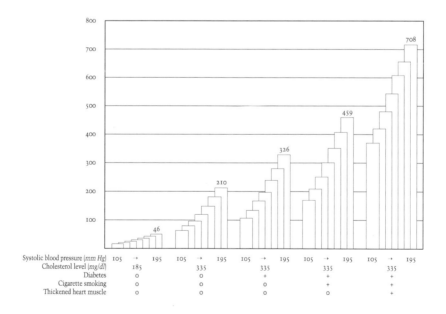

FIGURE I

Number of people per 1,000 who will develop coronary artery disease over an eight-year period related to the number of risk factors present in conjunction with various levels of blood pressure.

risks. Smoking, high blood pressure, and cholesterol will get plenty of their own space later on.

Table 1	
RISK FACTORS FOR CORONARY ARTERY DISEASE	
Those that can be changed (modifiable):	*Those that can't (non-modifiable):*
1. Smoking	1. Age
2. High blood pressure	2. Sex
3. Diabetes	3. Family history
4. High total and LDL cholesterol levels	
5. Low HDL levels	
6. Obesity (greater than 30% ideal body weight)	

Non-modifiable Risk Factors

Sex, family history, and age are non-modifiable risk factors. There are various means by which one can successfully look and feel more youthful, but moisturizers and plastic surgery will not prevent heart attacks. You will look younger when you arrive in the emergency department with chest pain, but this is a superficial advantage at best. Recognizing that modern surgery can change a man into a woman, I still consider sex to be a "non-modifiable" risk factor. Age is considered a risk factor because from birth until death, the older you are, the greater your risk of developing heart disease.

Men are much more likely to develop heart disease than women (figure 2). Simply being male is an independent cardiac risk factor. Men suffer from heart attacks an average of 20 years earlier than women. In the absence of risk factors, heart attacks are extremely uncommon in otherwise healthy women prior to menopause. After menopause, however, a woman's risk approaches that of a man's and equals it by age 75. In an era of increasing competition between the sexes, this is a race in which men and women would prefer to remain on the sidelines.

A family history of heart disease is a frequent source of worry for many people. When questioned about family history, patients often relate tales of nonspecific heart ailments in a 94-year-old great-grandparent. Though I would not wish to be mislabelled as callous, the health of dear old granny is of minimal if any relevance. A family history of cardiac disease is classified as a **major risk factor** only if a mother or sister had a heart attack, bypass surgery, or coronary angioplasty before the age of 65, or a father or brother suffered from any of these before the age of 55. There are multiple types of heart problems, and only a history of heart attacks, coronary angioplasty, or coronary bypass surgery is relevant. Not all the risk factors are of the same importance. The most important risk factor is family history, followed by tobacco, diabetes, high blood pressure, and lipids.

Emotions

A great deal of press has centred on the influence of emotional state on heart disease. One study showed that **depression** increased the chance of developing a heart attack fourfold. This was a prospective study, meaning that depressed patients without evidence of heart disease were followed for a number of years to see who developed it. They were followed figuratively and not "tailed," which would have made them depressed *and* paranoid.

Grief is also a risk factor. The danger of suffering a heart attack is increased 14-fold within 24 hours of a loved one's death. Though the risk remains higher for at least a month, it is never as high as within the first two days.

Environmental stresses can definitely precipitate heart attacks. **Anxiety** is associated with a higher risk. For example, heart attacks increase after earthquakes. The cardiac event rate in Israel went up after Iraqi Scud missile attacks during the Gulf War. Avalanches, hurricanes, typhoons, floods, locusts, lice, and other biblical catastrophes have yet to be studied.

Anger may also trigger a heart attack. Within two hours of an angry outburst, the chance is doubled.

The ability of these emotions to provoke a heart attack is dependent on the presence of **pre-existing** heart disease. In other words, you have to be leaning over the edge before you can be tipped into the canyon.

Doctors have actually studied the relationship between heart disease and deer-hunting. Hunters dramatically increase their heart rates and show signs of reduced blood flow to their heart during the hunt. (The effect on the health of the deer was even greater, especially when they were being gutted.)

Gambling also can be quite stressful (no kidding). In a three-and-a-half-year period, there were more than 700 cardiac arrests in Las Vegas casinos and just over 150 survivors. Those aren't very good odds. Whereas some casinos in Canada are equipped with on-site emergency medical care, American casinos are not. This may be due to fear of liability.

The most common time of the day for a heart attack is in the morning, within two or three hours of arising. The worst seasons are winter and spring. So don't get angry after the death of a loved one from an earthquake triggered by a morning missile attack in the middle of winter during deer-hunting season while gambling!

Despite all of this hubbub about emotions, most people have **no identifiable trigger** preceding their heart attack.

Obesity

Weight is intricately linked to diet. The more calories you eat and the less you shed, the higher the number on your scale. Obesity is a risk factor for heart disease and is defined

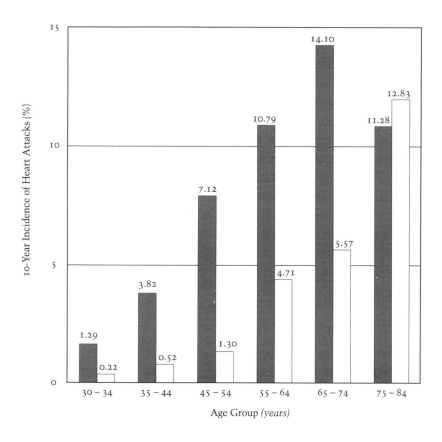

FIGURE 2

The likelihood of developing a heart attack depends on age and sex.
In this figure, men are represented in grey and women in white.
The data comes from over 5,000 people who were free of heart
disease at the beginning of the study and followed for 30 years.

by something called the **body mass index** (BMI). The BMI
relates weight to height, since the health of a 200-pound
person depends on whether she is under five feet tall or over
six feet tall. The BMI is calculated by taking your weight in
kilograms and dividing it by your height in metres squared.
So if you weigh 70 kilograms and are 1.8 metres tall, your
BMI is 21.6(70/1.8 x 1.8). A BMI over 27 defines obesity. A
BMI over 23 increases the risk of a heart attack. A person

who is 5'6" and weighs 154 pounds has a BMI of 25. The bottom line is that if you are overweight, you probably know it without having to learn the metric system.

Homocysteine

Homocysteine is not a fossil remnant of early man discovered by archaeologists, but rather an **amino acid**. Amino acids are the building blocks of proteins, like pieces of Lego. It has recently been discovered that high blood levels of homocysteine are a risk factor for the development of coronary artery disease. How important it is remains to be determined.

High homocysteine levels arise from a weakness in the body's ability to break it down into smaller pieces. The higher the level, the greater the risk. Unfortunately, there is no standard way to measure homocysteine levels, so results differ depending on how the measurement is done. Patients with coronary disease who have none of the usual risk factors, such as smoking and high lipids, could have high homocysteine levels. It may account for 5-10% of all deaths from coronary artery disease.

There are various causes for "hyperhomocysteinemia" (there has got to be an easier term!). Levels are partially determined by genetics, increase with age, and are higher in men than women, especially if the women are pre-menopausal. They are higher in smokers (as if they don't have enough trouble) and coffee drinkers. Carnivores, meaning meat-eaters, have higher levels than vegetarians. The more fruits and veggies we eat, the healthier the homocysteine. Who should have their blood homocysteine measured? There is no clear consensus on this point. Patients with a strong family history of premature coronary disease are good candidates, as are younger patients with heart disease and no major risk factors, but we are only just beginning to define homocysteine as a risk factor.

Folic acid, a B vitamin, lowers homocysteine levels when taken as a pill. Dosages of one, five, and 10 milligrams have been used. No study has ever looked at its benefits in reducing the incidence of coronary disease, so it is just too early to tell whether supplemental folate is useful. Vitamin B12 and vitamin B6 (pyridoxine) also lower high levels of homocysteine. If I had high levels of homocysteine, however, I would take folate supplements. I would also stuff myself with bushels of fruits and vegetables.

POINTS TO REMEMBER

- Risks for developing coronary artery disease that are non-modifiable include age, sex, and family history.

- The major risk factors for coronary artery disease that can be changed are smoking, high blood pressure, diabetes, high lipids, and obesity.

- Emotions such as depression, grief, anger, and anxiety may provoke a heart attack, but only if there is pre-existing disease in the blood vessels of the heart (coronary arteries).

- Heart attacks are more likely in the early morning hours and in the spring and winter.

- High blood levels of homocysteine increase the risk of a heart attack. Though folate reduces high levels, it remains to be seen whether this will reduce the risk of heart attacks.

3

ANATOMY OF
THE HEART

Coronary artery disease causes heart attacks. Learning how the heart works is a prerequisite to understanding this common condition. The heart is like a house with four rooms, two on the right side and two on the left (figure 3). The rooms with thick walls are called ventricles. The other two thinner rooms are called **atria** (singular = atrium). Each side of the heart (the left and the right) has one atrium and one ventricle. The rooms on the right (one ventricle and one atrium) connect to each other via a large door, which acts as a valve. The rooms on the left do the same. The right and left sides are not in direct contact with each other, but they do share walls. The larger and thicker-walled rooms (ventricles) propel blood to the body and lungs while the smaller ones (atria) act as reservoirs, storing the blood until it is sent into the ventricles.

Imagine the front door of the **left side** of the house opens onto a race track. People with arms full of food taken from the kitchen go out the front door and sprint around the track. As they run, they drop off the food for the spectators. Near exhaustion, they arrive at the back door on the **right side** of the house. They come in, then go through the front door on the **right side** to the kitchen. After loading up with more food, they go through the back door on the **left side** of the house and the cycle continues.

How in the world does such poor urban planning relate to the heart? The groceries represent oxygen and the kitchen represents the lungs. Blood full of nourishing oxygen is pumped to the body to meet the demands of everyday life. When the oxygen-poor blood returns to the heart, it is pumped to the lungs for oxygen replenishment. It then travels back to the heart and the cycle continues.

The doors represent heart valves and everyone has four of them. Heart valves control blood flow from the atria to the ventricles, and from the left ventricle and right ventricle to the body and lungs respectively. By definition, a valve only allows movement one way, so people can only move through the house in a single direction. Once the food has been gathered, there is no going back for seconds unless you finish the course. Like a house, the heart has an electrical wiring system in its walls. The surges of electricity are very regular, and each one activates a heartbeat. With each heartbeat, blood pulses through the rooms and valves (figure 3).

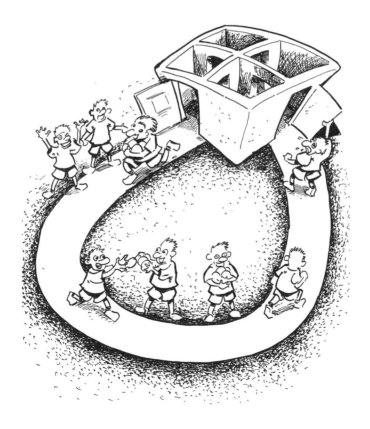

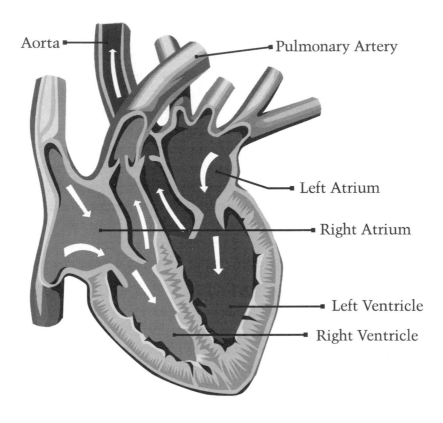

Aorta

Pulmonary Artery

Left Atrium

Right Atrium

Left Ventricle

Right Ventricle

FIGURE 3

How does the heart receive the energy it requires to deliver blood to the body? It cannot simply rely on absorbing oxygen through the walls as blood moves through the chambers. The heart needs its own plumbing system. The plumbing system of the heart is the **coronary arteries**. These arteries are the tubes through which blood flows to nourish the heart with oxygen-rich blood. Arteries are found in every organ. Almost all of the blood which passes through the front door of the left side is propelled forward to the body. Immediately after passing through the front door, however, some of it is diverted into a tunnel system which courses through the walls of the heart like plumbing pipes. It is through this plumbing system that the first rush of people are shunted. Instead of dashing around the track, they travel through the network within the walls, supplying the heart muscle with nutrition.

Coronary artery disease, or CAD, causes heart attacks. It is the most common cause of death in North America. Statistics don't often affect us because the numbers are too large to comprehend in a personal way. There is nothing personal about a number. Approximately one million people suffer heart attacks in the United States per year. Roughly one quarter of these people die. More than half of these deaths occur suddenly before the person has reached a hospital, usually within three hours of first noticing symptoms. Many conclusions may be drawn from these simple facts. Those that deserve special emphasis are:

- If you have symptoms of a heart attack, don't allow denial to delay your visit to the hospital. Many people die with an antacid in their stomachs, having incorrectly attributed their symptoms to indigestion. Many others try to sleep it off, never to wake up.

- For many individuals and their families, there is no second chance.

Coronary Arteries & Heart Attacks

As mentioned, the heart receives blood from its own pipes, which are called coronary arteries. Every artery in the body has a name. This dates from the earliest days of medicine when the motto was, "We don't know what it does, but let's name it." The brain, for example, receives blood through cerebral arteries, while the kidneys are served by the renal arteries. The anatomy of the coronary arteries (figure 4) is easy to understand when a tree analogy is used (figure 5). The coronary arteries are like branches of a tree that deliver water and minerals to the leaves. The leaves represent the individual muscle cells of the heart which

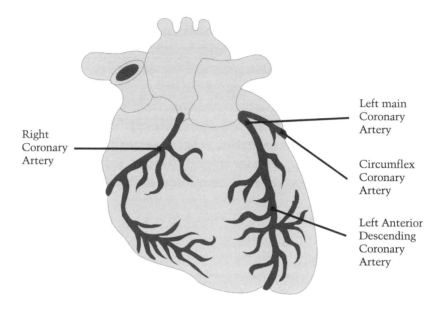

Right
Coronary
Artery

Left main
Coronary
Artery

Circumflex
Coronary
Artery

Left Anterior
Descending
Coronary
Artery

FIGURE 4

contract during a heartbeat. There is a left coronary system and a right coronary system. Each individual tree is closely intertwined with the other. The left coronary system almost always supplies a greater amount of heart muscle than the right, so coronary disease in the left side usually causes more damage. Narrowings and heart attacks may occur anywhere in the coronary tree.

The right system is called the **right coronary artery**, or RCA for short. It is one big blood vessel with various branches. In some people, the size of the branches may be very large. These branches may merit special attention if narrowings are discovered. The left side is more complex. The origin of the left system is called the **left main** and it quickly divides into two major arteries. They are called the **left anterior descending artery**, almost always referred to as the LAD, and the **circumflex artery**, known as the "**circ**." As with the right side, the branches can be very large and important and they have their own names. The most important thing

to remember about coronary arteries and heart attacks is
that there is a critical distinction between a **narrowing**
and a **complete obstruction**. Narrowings of the left main
are called "widow makers." So much heart muscle relies on
blood flow through this segment that a complete obstruction of the left main is almost certain death.

If we return to our tree, imagine that the water supply
is suddenly interrupted by a blockage within one of the
branches. If that were to occur, then the part of the tree
nourished by that particular branch would die. It would not
necessarily die immediately. After a few hours, the leaves
would become lifeless. After a few weeks, only shrivelled
remnants would be attached to the branches. If a similar
event happens in the heart, it is called a **heart attack**. A heart
attack (also known as a **coronary**, a **myocardial infarction**,

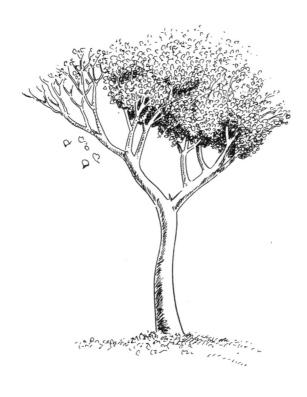

FIGURE 5

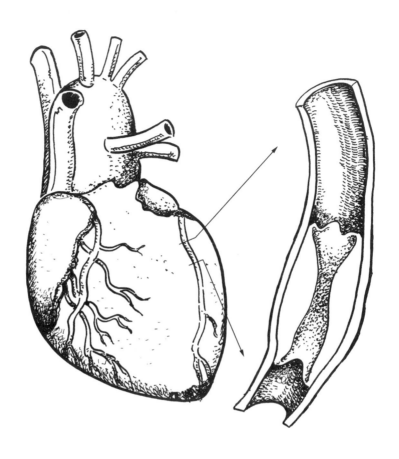

FIGURE 6
Cross section of a fat deposit lining the wall of a
coronary artery, shown in enlarged section.
The resultant narrowing may cause a heart attack.

and an **MI**) means that **blood flow to a part of the heart stops due to a blood clot within one of the coronary arteries**. Blood clots are gelatinous blobs and are far more likely to form within an already narrowed artery. Therefore, narrowings (due to fat deposits called **atherosclerosis**) place people at a greater risk of suffering from a heart attack (figure 6).

An obstruction in the water supply to a portion of the tree does not necessarily result in the death of the entire tree. The tree's overall well-being is dependent on many things. The most important variable is where the obstruction occurs, or, put another way, how much of the tree is affected by the blockage of flow. If the flow of water is obstructed at the very base of the tree, as when a chainsaw slices through it, then the entire tree dies. If only the uppermost branches are affected by a blockage near the top of the tree, the damage may go unrecognized and the tree will continue to function normally.

The heart behaves in much the same manner. A heart attack affecting only a small branch near the end of a blood vessel may have little, if any, effect on a patient. A blockage near the **origin** of one of the coronary arteries, however, will usually cause severe damage to a large portion of heart muscle, or death. People who survive such "massive" heart attacks are often left with terrible symptoms of heart failure, because such a large amount of their heart dies. They are fatigued by the slightest exertion and may develop shortness of breath walking from the bedroom to the kitchen.

A heart attack is defined as the death of heart muscle. It will no more regain normal function than your hand would if a few fingers were crushed. That area of the heart that previously housed healthy muscle becomes a home to functionless scar tissue, with the same components as a scar on your skin.

Bradycardia

Some areas of the heart have very specialized functions and they all depend on blood for normal operation. The heart has a generator which sends out electrical currents. This ensures order and regularity of the heartbeat. If the blood vessel responsible for nourishing this generator is involved in a heart attack, a deadly scenario may occur: the heartbeat may become dangerously slow and the heart may be left without a conductor. This is called **bradycardia**, and it can be dangerous enough to cause death. The muscle may eventually stop beating, like a dog waiting for direction from its master. The lesson here is that all heart attacks, no matter how small, can be deadly.

Ventricular Tachycardia

Any injury, whether at the top or bottom of the tree, creates a potentially unstable environment in the heart muscle. What do I mean by instability? The damaged area, like all heart muscle, has an electrical current passing through it which originates in the electrical generator. The electricity may shortcircuit when blood flow is interrupted. If this happens, the walls may generate their own electrical current, which rapidly spreads like a wave throughout the entire muscle. The damaged area continues to send wave upon wave of electrical pulses like infantrymen over the tops of bunkers. Each wave represents a heartbeat. This creates such a rapid heart rate that death suddenly occurs because the heart just cannot pump that fast. This common and deadly rhythm is called **ventricular tachycardia**. Right now, your heart beats probably anywhere from 40 to 100 times per minute, depending on what you're doing. Imagine that it beats 250 times or more. Clearly this would not be sustainable for long. Ultimately, the heart simply stops.

CK

One of the ways a heart attack can be diagnosed in the hospital involves the death of heart muscle cells (called **myocytes**). When the myocytes die from lack of blood flow, they burst and their cell contents are released into the surrounding tissue. Eventually, these proteins and cell remnants are absorbed into the bloodstream where they can be measured by a simple blood test. It's as if a million tiny confetti-filled balloons exploded. The amount of "confetti" measured in the blood gives an early approximation of the amount of damage to the heart. If a person complains of chest pain but the "blood confetti level" is normal, then a heart attack can be virtually excluded. The name of the confetti is **creatinine kinase**, abbreviated as CK by doctors. A normal baseline level of CK is always circulating in the blood. It comes from sources other than the heart, such as your muscles. Any rise in the CK accompanied by chest pain necessitates a confirmatory blood test to diagnose whether the source of the elevation is heart muscle. A more specific test which is only recently being used to diagnose a heart attack, measures **troponin**, which comes only from myocytes.

Congestive Heart Failure

Congestive heart failure, or CHF, is the result of heart fatigue. The heart muscle is extremely resistant to fatigue during our lifetime. It has to be or it couldn't generate the two and a half to three billion heartbeats needed to carry you into your seventies. When a significant chunk of heart muscle is destroyed from a coronary obstruction too close to the "base of your tree," the heart can no longer meet the needs of the body and the blood isn't pumped forward as vigorously. It's as if two assembly-line workers were on a shift and one fell asleep. If the conveyor belt continued to deliver work for two, then the assembly line would start to back up. That is exactly what the blood does: it backs up and fluid seeps into the lungs, since this is where the oxygen-rich blood is delivered from. This scenario describes congestive heart failure. The first symptoms are fatigue and shortness of breath both when lying flat and/or when exerting oneself.

Angina

Now that you have a fundamental understanding of what a heart attack is, angina becomes an easier concept to grasp. In its most elementary form, **angina** is a sensation of pain or pressure due to narrowings in the coronary arteries.

There are two important caveats. Firstly, angina is not always pain. When asked about chest pain, patients will frequently deny that they suffer from it.

"What about your history of heart attacks?" I ask.

"Well, that was more a feeling of discomfort," they reply. The point is that angina can manifest as a myriad of different sensations, including pain, pressure, heat, heartburn, indigestion, upset stomach, numbness, twitch, tickle, etc. If your experience does not include any of these symptoms, that does not mean your symptoms are not angina. There are as many descriptions as there are patients. At times, the history will be so classic that the diagnosis of angina is never in doubt. More often, however, the story is vague and atypical and the heart cannot be excluded as the source of discomfort.

The second feature of angina meriting emphasis is its location. Though the classic description is central chest discomfort radiating down the left arm, there are many potential variations. I have seen patients with nothing but numbness in the fingertips, jaw pain, throat discomfort, and even a toothache. Angina may manifest as back pain or abdominal pain. Because of such variability in symptoms and location, more objective tests such as **electrocardiograms** (ECGs) and **exercise treadmill exams** are used to diagnose coronary disease.

Angina arises when the heart needs more blood to do its job than the coronary arteries can supply. Angina occurs in people who have severe narrowings in their coronary arteries. Heart attacks occur when the blood flow is **completely blocked**.

At rest, the blood supply to the heart is adequate to meet its needs. The heart is more of a servant than a master, however, and the body controls the reins. When the body needs more blood during exertion or stress, the heart is put on a treadmill it cannot get off. It must pump faster and harder, which requires more blood and oxygen for the heart muscle. When one decides to walk, jog, climb stairs, or have sex (especially on stairs), the body flogs the heart into pumping out more blood. If the heart cannot supply itself with enough blood for the job, it starts complaining and crying for you to stop. This is angina. It's an effective early warning system. The symptoms of angina are due to insufficient blood supply. This is similar to your legs fatiguing during a jog, or your arms screaming as you attempt one more repetition of a weight. If you continue to push yourself during angina, you risk suffering a heart attack.

Coronary narrowings, known generically as **lesions**, are not static. With time they progress, and less blood is able to squeeze through to supply the heart. It subsequently takes less and less activity to cause angina. Twenty minutes of symptom-free tennis becomes five minutes before the onset of chest pain (or pressure, or dullness, or tension, etc.). Some patients get angina once a week while others may suffer from multiple episodes per day. Emotional upset, which may raise heart rate and blood pressure, is a frequent cause of angina. In patients with stable and predictable symptoms of angina, a nitroglycerin tablet or spray taken a few minutes before the activity will often prevent the episode.

Patients are often confused by the sudden appearance of angina. The following analogy helps explain why the onset of symptoms reflects a **continuum**, and not the **sudden** development of coronary disease. A village situated on the river depends on it for food. Though the fishermen catch 100 fish per day, 1,000 fish swim by during that time. When visitors arrive, the fishermen easily double their catch to 200 fish. If the river progressively narrowed upstream (let's say there was a chemical plant dumping toxic sludge along

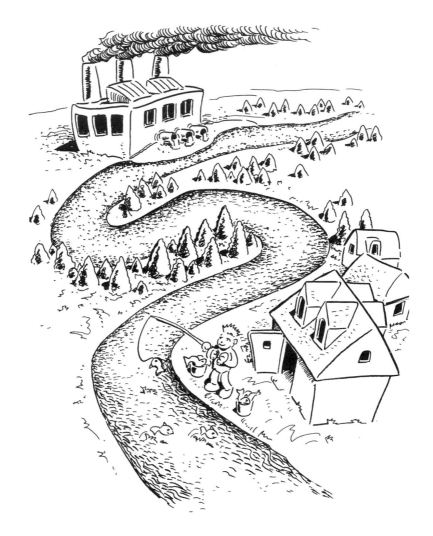

the banks), allowing fewer and fewer fish to pass by, the villagers would be oblivious to the change until less than 100 fish swam by (or if there were visitors, less than 200). Even if there was a 50% decline, they would still be able to feed their families. The coronary arteries work in exactly the same way. During rest, there may be progressive narrowing from atherosclerotic sludge. This remains unrecognized until the encroachment on flow becomes critical (less than 100 fish), or until more blood flow (more than 200 fish) is required.

Angina is defined as stable or unstable. Stable angina implies that it is infrequent, predictable, and of short duration. Most cardiac patients have stable angina. Unstable angina means that the pattern of the angina has **changed**. It may be occurring with increasing frequency or duration. Any symptom of angina within a month of a heart attack is by definition **unstable**. Patients with unstable symptoms should immediately be seen in a hospital.

With the onset of angina, the first move is to stop whatever activity has caused it and rest. In many people, the chest pain will gradually resolve within a variable amount of time, say five to 10 minutes. In others, a nitroglycerin spray or tablet will be required to stop the pain. Nitroglycerin dilates the coronary arteries, making them wider. So instead of a compact car fitting through the tunnel, an entire tractor-trailer gets in. It also dilates the blood vessels to the head, which explains why headaches are a common side effect. If three sprays or tablets of nitroglycerin spaced about three to five minutes apart do not relieve the angina, then you should make a beeline for the nearest hospital. The angina may actually be a heart attack, and **the greatest period of instability is the first few hours**. If your angina is more severe than usual, occurs at rest, or is associated with significant sweating or shortness of breath, one hand should be reaching for nitroglycerin while the other moves for the phone.

Denial

One reason so many people die of heart attacks prior to reaching hospital is denial. Their last words are often "It's only a little indigestion." Waiting for the inning to finish or for dessert to arrive are poor excuses for neglecting potentially serious symptoms. Denial is reflected in a stubborn refusal to admit there may be a problem. Many patients only come to the hospital at the insistence of their spouse. If the chest pain is from a heart attack, then drugs exist which can smash open the blockage and re-establish blood flow to the heart. Administered early, these drugs are effective and can save your life. Heart damage can be **prevented** if treatment is started early. Patients who arrive at the hospital soon after the onset of symptoms have the best chance for recovery. There is a narrow window of opportunity. I have treated many people whose hearts stopped within minutes of their arrival in the emergency department. If they had waited a little longer to call the ambulance, they would be dead. **When it comes to heart attacks, delay equals death.** Whereas a heart attack results in the death of heart tissue, angina is a warning symptom that such damage can occur. A patient may arrive at the hospital complaining of angina. If there is subsequent evidence of heart damage (remember the confetti?), the diagnosis the doctor makes changes from **angina** to **myocardial infarction**.

This chapter has provided a foundation from which to alter your lifestyle. In the short time it has taken to read this, you have acquired fundamental information to live healthier and longer. As you continue on, you will be amazed at the knowledge you gain, and with it the confidence to implement change.

POINTS TO REMEMBER

- **The heart has four rooms (two atria and two ventricles), four doors (valves), a plumbing system (the coronary arteries), and electrical wiring.**

- **If enough heart muscle is destroyed by a heart attack, congestive heart failure results. Its prognosis can be worse than that of most cancers.**

- **Narrowings in a coronary artery cause angina, a warning for a heart attack. Complete blockage of a coronary artery causes a heart attack.**

- Angina is not always pain and does not always occur in the chest. Because heart problems produce many atypical symptoms, they should always be treated seriously and further testing is often required to establish the diagnosis.

- Denial can kill you.

4

LIPID LEVELS

At present, there are only four routinely performed lipid tests: **total cholesterol**, LDL, HDL, and **triglycerides**. Collectively, they represent the **lipid profile** (table 2). This section will provide information about what these tests measure and what desirable levels are. You should finish this chapter with knowledge of the blood lipid levels safest for you and your heart. Alternatively, you could leave this business to your doctor and simply follow his or her advice. As you will discover, though, the information is simple and concise. Knowing your target will help you realize your goals. The ramifications of having slightly high lipid levels are very different than if they were three times the normal level.

Atherosclerosis

When cholesterol deposits itself in the walls of coronary arteries, the result is called **atherosclerosis**, or hardening of the arteries. These areas of cholesterol buildup are known as **plaques**, or more generically, **lesions**. Cholesterol deposits are like debris and garbage in a sewage system accumulating in the walls of the drainage pipes. As more and more layers of crud build up, the flow of waste becomes progressively restricted until the pipes no longer function as effective conduits. As outlined previously, when blood flow is blocked in one of the coronary arteries from progressive atherosclerosis, a heart attack occurs. There are many factors involved in cholesterol accumulation in coronary arteries, and high blood cholesterol levels is a major risk. The higher the blood cholesterol level, the more likely it will deposit in the walls and cause a heart attack.

Fats & Lipids

Fat and lipid are the same thing. Though they are synonymous terms, lipid has a more scientific flavour and is the preferred word for the medical community. **Cholesterol** is a type of lipid just as a Cadillac is a type of car. Other kinds of lipids include **triglycerides** and certain **vitamins** (A, D, E, K, and beta-carotene). What distinguishes lipids from other molecules in the body is their insolubility in blood. This means they will not dissolve. Therefore, lipids such as cholesterol require a special means of transportation through the bloodstream to carry out their daily jobs. They travel around on the blood superhighway in special vehicles called **lipoproteins**.

Table 2

LIPID PROFILE

1. Total Cholesterol
2. LDL
3. HDL
4. Triglycerides

Lipoproteins (LDL & HDL)

Lipoproteins are like lipid taxicabs. Knowing the blood levels of these lipoproteins is very important in assessing heart disease risk. This is why a blood lipid screen includes not only cholesterol, but also LDL, HDL, and triglycerides.

Though there are many types of lipoproteins, the ones of

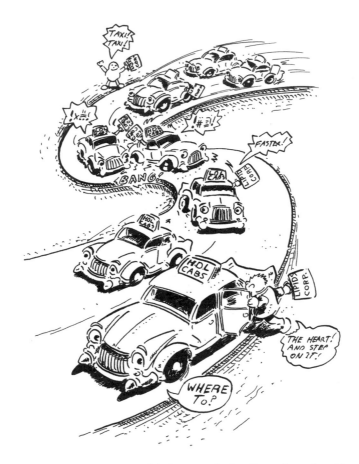

consequence are LDL, which stands for **low density lipoprotein**, and HDL, which is **high density lipoprotein**. LDL is known as the **bad cholesterol**. LDL is not actually cholesterol, but rather the back upon which cholesterol hitches a ride. As is true with high levels of cholesterol, high levels of LDL portend a greater risk of developing coronary artery disease. About 65% of cholesterol is transported in LDL, 25% in HDL, and the rest moves around in the other lipoproteins.

Cholesterol is an integral building block of cells and is involved in a variety of diverse physiologic events. It originates in the body from two sources: the liver which manufactures it, and the intestines which absorb it from the diet.

LDL transports cholesterol from the liver and intestines to the rest of the body. When excessive amounts of LDL travel through the arteries, they dump their cholesterol load into the arterial walls, creating **atherosclerotic lesions**. This is why a high level of LDL is bad for you. The higher the level, the more likely cholesterol will find a home in your arteries.

HDL is known as the **good cholesterol**. It has a reverse transport function. It ferries cholesterol **away** from the tissues, including the coronary arteries, and drops it off at the liver. Enzymes in the liver break down the cholesterol and it is used for energy. This is why high levels of HDL are good for you. The higher the HDL level, the more cholesterol gets carted away from the arteries for disposal by the liver. In fact, **a high level of HDL is more protective to the heart than a high level of LDL is dangerous**. Unfortunately the corollary is also true. A low HDL level is a very powerful risk factor for the development of coronary artery disease. Without sufficient HDL to carry cholesterol away, athero-sclerotic plaques grow. Measuring HDL is very important for establishing coronary risk. Factors which affect HDL are listed in table 3.

Table 3

HDL LEVELS

Decreased by	Increased by
1. Carbohydrate intake	1. Saturated fat intake
2. Obesity	2. Alcohol
3. Diabetes	3. Exercise
4. Polyunsaturated fat intake	4. Cholesterol intake
5. Cigarettes	
6. Beta blockers (a heart drug)	
7. Sedentary lifestyle	

Cholesterol levels vary with age and sex. This is not meant to imply that engaging in more sex will lower cholesterol, at least not directly. Levels rise with age. In very old age (your definition will likely depend on your birth date) lipid levels tend to **drop off** as sicker individuals with the higher cholesterol levels do the same, leaving only the healthiest people around. Cholesterol begins to increase in both sexes at the onset of puberty. Pre-menopausal women have lower levels compared to men of the same age until they reach their fifties, at which time women surpass their male counterparts. There are no significant differences in lipid levels between different races, though blacks tend to have marginally higher levels of the protective HDL. Healthy people, no matter what age, have lower blood lipids.

Acceptable lipid levels will differ depending on age, sex, and the presence of other cardiac risk factors. A 25-year-old woman with an LDL level of 4.1 mmol/L (expressed as 160 mg/dl in the U.S.) has so little risk of cardiac disease that no intervention would even be considered. However, a 60-year-old man with a previous heart attack and the same LDL level would be aggressively treated with diet and drugs due to the association of this value with more heart attacks. Mmol/L and mg/dl are units of measurement. They are quantities, like pounds or litres.

Testing

The first question to address is who should have their lipids checked. The answer is everyone over age 20. For those with a family history of premature coronary disease, age should not be a criterion for testing.

Measuring lipids requires patient preparation or else the results may be invalid. A full lipid panel, including total cholesterol, LDL, HDL, and triglycerides, requires a 14-hour fast and abstention from alcohol for three days to assure accuracy. If the lipid panel is normal, it should be repeated every three to five years. If abnormal, another lipid screen should be done to confirm the result before therapy is started. Levels may be invalid if there is a recent major weight change, dietary change, operation, or trauma. Cholesterol levels may be up to 10% higher during the winter and nobody knows why.

Lipid levels often fall after a heart attack or other serious illness and return to pre-illness values after three months. This does not mean that measuring them is inappropriate at the time of hospitalization, as they may still be abnormal and require therapy. For example, an LDL of 4.1 mmol/L (160 mg/dl) in a patient admitted with a heart attack should be lowered with drugs. All cardiac patients without prior knowledge of a recent (i.e., within six months) lipid profile who arrive at the hospital with a heart attack or angina should have their lipids measured.

Primary and Secondary Lipid Disorders

If no cause for an abnormal lipid profile can be identified, it is classified as a **primary** problem. If a causative disease is recognized, however, then the abnormality is called a **secondary** disorder. Patients should be aware of a number of simple tests used to exclude secondary causes of high lipids. Screening tests are important because if a disease is identified, treating it could correct the problem without having to use cholesterol-lowering medication. Tests your doctor should perform to exclude a cause for a high lipid level include **fasting blood sugar**, a TSH (thyroid-stimulating hormone), **creatinine** (a measure of kidney function, not the heart enzyme), a **urinalysis**, and **liver function tests** (AST, ALT, and ALP). Alcohol consumption should be reviewed as should a list of medications, as there are many drugs which can alter the lipid profile. Stopping the drug may correct the problem.

Some lipid disorders are transmitted through generations. This means that a parent can pass the condition to a child, resulting in the child developing heart problems due to very high lipid levels. It is thus important to identify genetic lipid problems early so that all relatives can be tested and treatment can be initiated quickly. There are a number of clues which point to a genetic cause of a lipid disorder. For example, a patient who develops the manifestations of coronary disease **prematurely** (at an early age) may have genetically high lipids. Lipid measurements should be performed in his or her siblings and children. Physical findings suggestive of a significant genetic component include lipid deposits in the skin, commonly on areas of the hands and feet (called **xanthomas**), and just under the eyes (called **xanthelasmas**). (These words may prove very useful in Scrabble games, or perhaps as names for twins.) Very high lipid levels, even in the absence of cardiac disease, may indicate a genetic cause. Values of particular concern are an LDL greater than 7.5 mmol/L (290 mg/dl), total cholesterol more than 8.5 (330), triglycerides above 10 (890), and HDL less than 0.6 (23).

The following definitions are useful (all values are expressed both in mmol/L and mg/dl):

LDL

under 3.36 (130) = normal

3.36–4.14 (130–160) = elevated

4.14 (160) = very elevated

TOTAL CHOLESTEROL

under 5.17 (200) = normal

5.17–6.18 (200–240) = elevated

6.18 (240) = very elevated

HDL

0.9–1.6 (35–60) = normal

TRIGLYCERIDES

under 2.26 (200) = normal

2.26–4.50 (200–400) = elevated

4.50–11.28 (400–1000) = moderately elevated

11.28 (1000) = very elevated

Interested parties (all of you reading this book) should be able to recite their lipid values as easily as height, weight, and the national anthem. What to do with these numbers is easy and depends on the presence of other cardiac risk factors. The first step is to identify the number of risk factors which apply to you from the following list:

RISK FACTORS FOR
CORONARY ARTERY DISEASE

1. Men over 45 years old
2. Women over 55 years old
3. Women under 55 years old who are post-menopausal and not on estrogen therapy
4. A family history of coronary artery disease in a father or brother before the age of 55 or a family history of coronary artery disease in a mother or sister before the age of 65
5. Cigarette use
6. High blood pressure or on medications for high blood pressure
7. Diabetes
8. HDL level less than 0.9 mmol/L (35 mg/dl)

How many risk factors do you have from the above list?

It is very encouraging when a patient expresses interest in modifying his or her cardiac risks. As I mentioned at the beginning of this section, attaining this goal is easier if there is a target to shoot for, so it's time to talk numbers. What levels are dangerous for which people?

The American College of Physicians (ACP) uses LDL as the linchpin to determine the overall approach. Some studies look at the **lipid ratio** in assessing cardiac risk. This refers to total cholesterol divided by HDL (TC/HDL). Though some doctors find the ratio useful, others only look at total cholesterol levels. I prefer to use a more detailed lipid analysis to determine risk and follow therapy. **When making treatment decisions, the most important number to look at is the LDL.** The LDL parallels the total cholesterol, so high levels of one suggest high levels of the other. Though many informed patients concentrate on their total cholesterol levels, the LDL is of greater importance in making decisions about risk and treatment. Some doctors recommend that total cholesterol be used to determine whether LDL should even be measured. I advocate measuring the entire lipid profile at the outset for all patients. Abnormal levels of HDL and triglycerides may also suggest the need for therapy independent of the LDL.

The following summary from the American College of Physicians highlights what lipid levels are right for you according to how many risk factors you have:

1. VERY HIGH RISK

If you have previously established coronary disease in the form of either *documented* angina, a heart attack, coronary angioplasty, or coronary surgery, your LDL should be under 2.6 (100). If you can achieve a lower LDL without medications, then more power to you. If your LDL is more than 3.4 (130), however, a dietary and drug approach should be undertaken simultaneously. The reason I specify *documented* angina is that many people complain of chest pain, but thankfully not all chest pain is angina.

2. HIGH RISK

Even in the absence of documented coronary artery disease, your risk of a heart attack can still be very high. If you have two or more of the above risk factors, your LDL should be under 3.4 (130). If it is more than 4.1 (160), dietary and drug therapy should be started immediately, instead of trying to reduce your LDL by diet alone. People with levels of 3.4 to 4.1 (130 to 160) can be tried on a diet for three months. If after three months the LDL is still above 3.4 (130), cholesterol-lowering drugs should be initiated.

3. LOW RISK

Less than two risk factors is considered a low risk. Though acceptable LDL levels are higher, they should still be under 4.1 (160). Anything more than 4.9 (190) in people with less than two risk factors should be treated with drugs and diet. Levels between 4.1 and 4.9 (160 and 190) can initially be dealt with by dietary modification alone, once again for a three-month period.

4. VERY LOW RISK

Men under 35 years of age and pre-menopausal women with less than two risks are considered **very** low risk, and LDL levels should be under 4.9 (190). An LDL between 4.9 and 5.7 (190 and 220) should be reduced with diet first and does not initially require drug therapy. Fewer Big Macs, more fruit. If above 5.7 (220), however, intervention is necessary with diet and drugs. Generally, pre-menopausal women have very low rates of coronary artery disease, even when their LDL and total cholesterol values are high. This is not true if there are other risk factors present.

A very high HDL (the "good" cholesterol) is considered a "negative" risk factor, meaning it counteracts and negates one other "positive" risk factor. Therefore if you have two risk factors and an HDL over 1.6 (60), you would actually be considered to have one risk factor.

This information is based on statistical data looking at the actual cardiac risk in all of these situations. Though I think this formula is appropriate for those in the very high and high risk categories, it may not properly address very high LDL levels in other groups. *Anyone* with an LDL level over 4.0 should pay close attention to dietary habits.

The American College of Physicians does not recommend drug therapy for isolated low levels of HDL (under 0.9 mmol/L or 35 mg/dl). If accompanied by another abnormal value — for example, elevated triglycerides — I would recommend drug therapy if diet and exercise are unsuccessful in correcting the abnormality. This recommendation does not have the same depth of scientific support as do the recommendations for high LDL levels.

Primary Prevention

A recent study from Scotland used a cholesterol-lowering medication in patients with no history of heart disease. This is called **primary prevention**, as it tries to stave off heart attacks instead of studying people who have already had them. These patients had LDL levels over 4.0 (about 160) and total cholesterol levels over 6.5 (about 250). The study showed a marked decrease in heart attacks and death in this population. This suggests that anyone between ages 45 and 64 with an LDL over 4.0 should be started on drugs and diet, even without other risks. The American College of Physicians' guidelines state that these patients should only be treated with drugs if there are two or more risk factors. Other researchers suggest that LDL levels in the low threes should be lowered with drugs. My position is in the middle. Though treating patients with LDL levels in the threes may gain momentum with further work, I advocate a drug approach if LDL remains above 4.0 despite diet and exercise, even if there are no other risks. For LDL levels below 4.0, it is reasonable to follow the ACP guidelines described above.

These new proposals by the authors of the Scottish study are a testament to the continuously evolving nature of lipid management. Their study is an example of the rapidly changing nature of medical practice. Recommendations on lipid management are shifting toward a more aggressive approach as new data becomes available. With ongoing lipid trials continuing worldwide, the recommendations proposed in this book may become obsolete, to be replaced by even more scientifically rigorous advice as new information emerges.

POINTS TO REMEMBER

- **The lipid profile is made up of total cholesterol, triglycerides, and two lipoproteins, called LDL and HDL.**

- **Cholesterol is a type of lipid (fat) which is transported in the blood by lipoproteins such as LDL and HDL.**

- **LDL is a bad lipoprotein which transports cholesterol to the arteries. HDL is a good lipoprotein which transports cholesterol away from the arteries.**

- **Lipid levels should be measured after a 14-hour fast with no alcohol use during the preceding three days to assure accuracy.**

- **The LDL level is the most important number unless one of the others is astronomically elevated, or in the case of HDL, very low.**

- **Acceptable lipid values depend on age and, most importantly, the presence or absence of other cardiac risk factors.**

- **Tabulate the number of risk factors you have, look at your lipid profile, put yourself into one of the four risk groups, and determine whether you need diet, drugs, both, or neither.**

- **An elevated HDL is a good risk factor and negates a bad risk factor.**

5

TRIGLYCERIDES & VLDL

Most dietary fat is in the form of **triglycerides**. They raise cholesterol and LDL levels through complex physiologic processes. (Using the phrase "complex physiologic processes" is a convenient way of saying I do not want to bore you with details.) Measured as part of the blood lipid profile, elevated triglycerides are the most common lipid abnormality. Triglycerides are stored in the body as fat, and are either used as a rapid source of energy in active people, or accumulate in all the wrong places on couch potatoes. Just as cholesterol is transported in blood by lipoproteins such as LDL and HDL, triglycerides are transported by a lipoprotein called **VLDL** (very low density lipoprotein). We do not routinely measure VLDL, since measuring triglycerides is a cheaper and equally effective means of gauging risk. Hypertriglyceridemia (medical lingo for abnormally high levels of triglycerides, with "hyper" meaning too much and "emia" meaning in the blood) is a risk factor for **pancreatitis**, a painful and dangerous inflammation of the pancreas.

High levels of **cholesterol** are unequivocally associated with an increased risk of coronary disease. The effect of high **triglycerides** on this risk is more controversial. High triglycerides are not as well accepted as high cholesterol as a risk factor for coronary artery disease, or CAD.

Only a minority of doctors claim that high tryglicerides are as important a risk as high cholesterol. Many studies have found that patients with heart disease are more likely to have high triglycerides, but when this data is rigidly subjected to statistical scrutiny, the link is too weak to stand up independently.

This does not mean there is no link between triglycerides and coronary disease. It suggests that the link is not very strong. While high triglycerides may still increase the likelihood of developing heart disease, it is not as likely to cause health problems as high cholesterol or a 12-gauge shotgun blast to the spleen.

Trials: Prospective and Retrospective

One reason that high triglycerides are not commonly thought of as a risk factor for CAD is the lack of prospective trials devoted to them. **Retrospective** trials look at events that have already happened. **Prospective** trials are designed to follow patients for the development of future events. The conclusions from retrospective studies lack teeth compared to prospective trials. The research into triglycerides is either retrospective or was not designed to look at the triglyceride question. The primary goal of this research was to determine the effect on cardiac health of lowering cholesterol, and triglyceride levels were an incidental measurement. To date, no study has been performed to specifically address whether lowering triglycerides as a **primary** intervention lowers the incidence of future heart disease. It is for this reason that advice about the benefits of lowering triglycerides cannot be dispensed with much scientific vigour.

Some genetic lipid disorders predispose individuals to early coronary artery disease. Sufferers are prone to heart attacks in their teens and twenties because of high blood lipids. All of the genetic conditions which raise cholesterol or LDL increase the risk of coronary disease. Other disorders selectively increase triglycerides. The enigma is that not all of the genetic disorders which raise triglyceride levels increase the risk of CAD. Though the relationship is unestablished, there remains much to be discovered. The link may yet be proven.

Who Is at Risk?

Until such scientific breakthroughs, what advice can be given to those with high triglycerides? Firstly, there are certain groups of patients who will lower their risk of heart disease by lowering triglyceride levels. There appears to be a gender difference, with women more at risk than men, especially women with diabetes, and patients who have low levels of HDL.

Table 4	
TRIGLYCERIDE LEVELS	
Increased by	*Decreased by*
1. Alcohol	1. Alcohol restriction
2. Diet high in carbohydrates	2. Exercise
3. Obesity	3. Weight loss
4. Diabetes	4. Low saturated fat diet
5. Medications	

Hypertriglyceridemia can be due to an assortment of causes (table 4). Alcohol intake will raise triglycerides. The more drunk you get, the larger the increase. It is also associated with a carbohydrate-rich diet. Industrialized nations owe their high triglycerides to excessive calories, invariably in the form of fat ("Would you like a diet cola with your burger and fries, sir?"). Overweight individuals and people with diabetes are more likely to have high triglycerides. Triglycerides may also be raised by some drugs, including estrogens, thiazide diuretics (used to treat high blood pressure), and certain beta-blockers (often used for high blood pressure and angina).

Reducing Your Triglycerides

Lowering triglycerides can be accomplished with a variety of simple interventions. It should be no surprise that regular exercise is one way to do it. Weight loss, perhaps not such a simple intervention, will improve high triglycerides as will moderating alcohol consumption and abstaining from cigarettes. A diet low in saturated fats may also lower levels, though this diet can be high in fatty fish such as salmon, tuna, and mackerel. I know what you're thinking: "What is there to live for if I can't partake of a few vices?" I believe that these bad habits can be broken. You must have the will and optimism to try and change them. It can be done. We are not talking about the split-second decision-making needed by a jet fighter pilot or when crossing a busy intersection. We are referring to decisions which can be gradually arrived at. Only you can make a difference in your own life and health.

Hypertriglyceridemia usually occurs in association with other lipid abnormalities. Lower those first and there will often be a beneficial spillover effect on triglyceride levels.

POINTS TO REMEMBER

- **Triglycerides are found in most dietary fats except for cholesterol.**

- **In most people, elevated triglyceride levels are not as major a risk for heart disease as high cholesterol.**

- **People with low levels of HDL and women with diabetes are at particular risk from high triglycerides and should be treated if other risk factors are present, though no good study has proven this.**

- Losing weight, exercising, and reducing alcohol are the best and cheapest ways to lower triglycerides (nobody said it was going to be easy).

6

DIET &
HEART DISEASE

Of all the cardiac risk factors, an excessive intake of fat is perhaps the most recognized yet least understood by the public. Given the ubiquitous presence of food in our lives and the obsessive behaviour it fosters, acquiring dietary knowledge is an effective means of improving cardiac health. Most people are aware of the need to reduce their fat intake. They merely lack sufficient knowledge and will-power to implement change. Simply cutting out **visible** fat, such as that present in beef, pork, and eggs, is inadequate. Many foods are saturated with invisible fats. The consumption of these fats must also be curtailed to have a positive impact on cardiac health. Because food pervades so much of our daily lives, it is a real challenge to alter eating habits. Controversies abound about the precise role dietary practices play in the development of heart disease. It is clear, however, that reducing fat intake decreases blood lipid levels. The lower these levels are, the less likely it is that coronary disease will develop.

The source of consumer information about diet is critically important. Misinformation by advertisers and special interest groups makes an inherently confusing subject even more difficult to understand. Despite claims to the contrary, it is not possible for the average Joe (or Josephine) to routinely consume a slab of beef, seven eggs, and a quarter pound of lean bacon and still maintain normal levels of blood cholesterol. Lean bacon is an oxymoron, reminiscent of "jumbo shrimp," "fresh frozen vegetables," and "real imitation cowhide." Bacon and sausage are cesspools of unhealthy ingredients. They are teeming with a vertiginous collection of fat and salt. Though I advocate dietary moderation, foods such as these should only be consumed by people who are terminally ill or aspire to be.

I could spew out simplistic advice about foods to avoid and foods to embrace, but that would be far less effective than providing a rationale for healthier nutritional practices. Standing on a pulpit of fruits and vegetables, urging the populace to abandon unsafe dietary habits, is unlikely to change eating behaviour. This section includes simple information about a heart-healthy diet. It also includes samples of important scientific data upon which nutritional advice is based. My purpose is not to furnish an exhaustive review of the world of nutrition. The focus of this book is heart disease, not cancer, headaches, or immune disorders. My intent is to supply people with effective dietary guidance. Used properly, this information will decrease your likelihood of developing coronary artery disease and possibly limit its progression. This is not homeopathic advice. It is scientific. You should eat vegetables, not bathe in them (unless you're bathing in them for personal reasons, of course).

The complexity of science can be intimidating. As a result, most people avoid it. I do not expect this chapter will motivate you to pursue a Ph.D. in lipid biochemistry. It is a more practical educational tool. There are no assurances that following my recommendations will guarantee health. There are people who die from heart attacks despite reasonably sane dietary habits and reasonably normal blood cholesterol readings. This is because the development of coronary artery disease is a complex interplay of various elements, some of which are known and others that await discovery. Some of these elements simply cannot be altered. The situation is analogous to gambling. Holding three of a kind in a poker hand does not assure you of winning money. There are a number of uncontrollable variables which can still deny you the victory. Following advice about diet (and the other cardiac risk factors) is tantamount to holding three of a kind. Your odds are improved, but there are no promises of success. Nonetheless, I would rather have three queens than a pair of aces. As you continue to absorb and implement nutritional information, your hand (and heart) will become stronger and stronger. It has been proven that planning your diet with sound nutritional advice promotes weight loss, improves blood pressure, and lowers cholesterol.

Framingham, MR FIT, Seven Countries', & The African Savannah

In matters of illness and health, conclusions must be proven and not simply surmised. This is in the best interest of patients seeking answers in a complex field. For example, if I tell you that the surest way to fight heart disease is to make a necklace from the kneecaps of African hummingbirds, then before going to the expense and trouble, you should expect this advice to be scientifically validated. I should be able to provide you with a study describing hundreds or thousands of people who trampled the Serengeti with gun holsters around their waists and waited in tall grass to blow the stuffing (though hopefully not the kneecaps) out of the first hummingbird to show its sorry little body. I should provide you with reams of statistics demonstrating less heart disease in people wearing hummingbird kneecap necklaces. Where are we otherwise? In the medieval domain of shysters and charlatans, who are more interested in maintaining their bank accounts than improving your health. I caution you to be wary of smooth-talking hucksters trumpeting remedies for your ills. If it cannot be proven, then it may not be true; it is only a belief, no different from any other cultural mythology. I would be happy to wear a garland of kneecaps, but I will only do so when the claim of their effectiveness is elevated from the depths of **belief** to the heights of **proof**. Making a suggestion based solely on belief is common. Physicians dispense stacks of medical advice that is yet to be adequately proven. The difference is that it should be espoused as belief, not dressed up as fact. It is easy to make an arbitrary health claim. It is markedly more difficult and time-consuming to prove it. Why the tangent? I'll briefly explain how doctors have arrived at the conclusion that high cholesterol is bad for you.

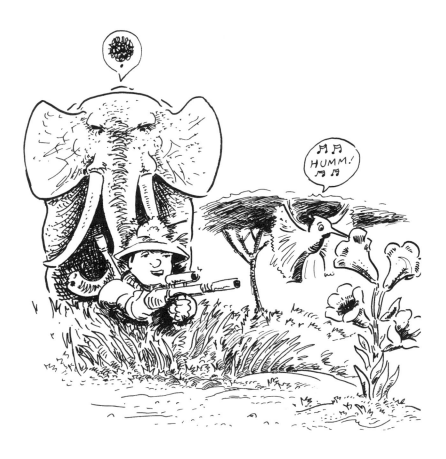

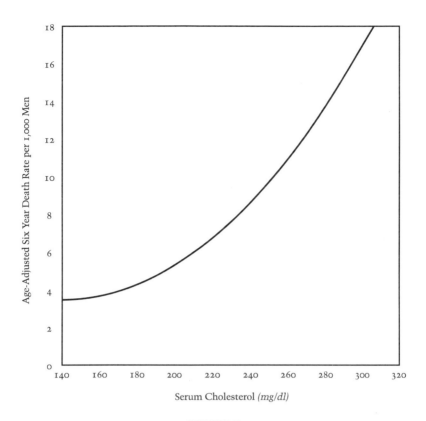

FIGURE 7

Relation of serum cholesterol to death caused by coronary artery disease in men 35 to 57 years of age during an average follow-up of six years. The risk increased steadily, particularly above levels of 200 mg/dl.

The relationship between cholesterol and coronary artery disease was definitively established in a series of important epidemiologic studies. Epidemiology is the study of the factors which cause disease (i.e., lipids) and the disease itself (i.e., coronary artery disease). It looks at such relationships statistically in complex ways. Epidemiology quantifies the chance of developing AIDS from unprotected sex and informs smokers of the precise risk of acquiring lung cancer. Boring but very important.

An example of one such study is the **Framingham Heart Study**, probably the most important cardiac trial ever. It was started in 1948 and is still ongoing, following the lives (and blood) of thousands of people from Framingham, Massachusetts. Among its important and unassailable conclusions is that **the higher the level of LDL, and the lower the HDL, the greater the chance of developing coronary artery disease. What we now accept as fact took years of carefully controlled observations to prove.**

MR FIT (Multiple Risk Factor Intervention Trial) is another important heart study. It confirmed the Framingham results (figure 7) and showed that the lower the cholesterol, the lower the risk of developing coronary artery disease. The study also demonstrated that at any given level of cholesterol, the older you are, the greater the risk. Therefore, a 60-year-old with a cholesterol of 6.7 has a higher chance of developing heart problems than a 40-year-old with the same cholesterol.

The final study in this trio is the **Seven Countries' Study**, which demonstrated that the presence of coronary artery disease varies in different parts of the world. The lowest incidence was found in Japan and the former Yugoslavia. The highest was in Eastern Finland where the chance of developing a fatal heart attack was 14 times higher than in Japan. In this trial, the countries whose citizens had the highest cholesterol levels had the highest death rates from CAD. Countries with the lowest cholesterol levels had the fewest deaths from CAD. The cardiovascular death rates for 34 different countries are listed in table 5.

But how do we know that cholesterol levels are related to the dietary practices of a given culture? Why not simply attribute the findings to genetics or astrological charts? Maybe coronary risk is actually determined by planetary motion. Perhaps high cholesterol only occurs in people born under the sign Libra (I hope not!). Associations such as those presented above have inherent biases. It would be like saying that most people who get into car accidents are wearing shoes, so shoes must be responsible for the accidents.

Table 5

CARDIOVASCULAR MORTALITY
FOR MEN & WOMEN AGES 35–74

	Men (per 100,000)	Women (per 100,000)
Russia	1015	493
Hungary	984	454
Bulgaria	912	487
Poland	899	392
Romania	895	526
Czech Republic	855	375
Scotland	655	325
Argentina	651	302
Northern Ireland	628	286
Finland	622	217
Ireland	618	259
England/Wales	516	234
New Zealand	499	230
Germany	493	214
Norway	486	180
Austria	476	207
United States	475	226
Denmark	470	206
Sweden	451	171
Puerto Rico	439	226
Portugal	422	217
Netherlands	417	169
Greece	413	214
Israel	397	231
China	387	281
Belgium	387	173
Australia	374	172
Canada	369	158
Italy	341	153
Switzerland	338	124
Spain	312	145
Mexico	294	206
France	260	118
Japan	234	95

This important question was addressed in a landmark study which looked at the presence of coronary artery disease in Japanese men living in Japan, Hawaii, and San Francisco. Because they were all Japanese, their genetic background was the same, and therefore results could not be explained by genetic differences. The dietary habits of each group reflected the area in which they lived. This addressed a criticism of the Seven Countries' Trial, where it was said that the genetic makeup of each country was so diverse, the differences in coronary disease may have had nothing to do with diet, but rather were a reflection of different genes. (There was no documentation of their astrological signs.)

The result of this latest trial was interesting. In Japan, where the diet is low in fat, the incidence of coronary disease was low. In Hawaii, where the fat intake was somewhere between Japan and the rest of the United States, there was more coronary disease. On the mainland (San Francisco), where the fat intake among Japanese was as high as that of other Americans, the rate of coronary artery disease was highest. Since all participants in the trial had the same genetic background, a dietary link in the development of coronary disease was proven.

The more fat eaten, the more likely a person will develop the problem. This result does not minimize the importance of genetics. It simply reinforces that there are additional factors such as diet which have an impact on the development of CAD. Countries where vegetarianism is common have much less coronary artery disease than countries where meat is a religion. In Asia, which has traditionally had low rates of coronary disease, the adoption of a more Westernized diet full of "fast food" is resulting in dramatic increases in the number of heart attacks.

Diet & Cholesterol

The meat of the next chapter relates to dietary advice. Before we get to this, it is worth considering the basis for our doctrine that **lowering** fat intake lowers cholesterol and coronary artery disease. The previous discussion established the link between high fat intake, high cholesterol levels, and coronary disease. However, we still have not shown that lowering fat intake is beneficial, and it would be irresponsible to simply assume this. People need proof that eating less fat will favourably alter their lipid profile and reduce their chances of succumbing to a heart attack. So why have physicians decided to advise patients to lower their cholesterol levels with diet and/or drugs?

The answer lies with numerous studies involving thousands of patients. In these so-called **dietary intervention trials**, large populations of people were divided into two groups. One group ate a low fat diet and the other consumed a regular diet. Among the conclusions were the following:

1. Low fat diets lower cholesterol levels and this is associated with less coronary artery disease.

2. Low fat diets may prevent progression of already established coronary artery disease.

3. People on low fat diets have fewer heart attacks and less angina.

Multiple studies have closely examined the effect of lipid-lowering medications on heart disease.

Suffice it to say that **lowering blood cholesterol by diet and/or drugs reduces coronary artery disease**. Reducing fat intake is difficult because it usually involves a tremendous alteration of deeply ingrained eating habits. Most people would be surprised by the different foods that contain unhealthy fat. The next section includes a description of the sources of healthy and unhealthy fats in our food.

POINTS TO REMEMBER

- **"Invisible fats" play a major role in raising cholesterol.**

- **The higher your blood levels of cholesterol and LDL, the greater your chance of having a heart attack.**

- The more fat you consume, the higher your blood levels of cholesterol and LDL will be.

- The risk of a heart attack is reduced by lowering blood cholesterol and LDL through dietary fat reduction and drugs.

- Hummingbird kneecaps make a nice garland but do nothing for your cardiac health.

7

FOOD &
HEART DISEASE

There are innumerable books which simply list the **precise** nutritional makeup of every obscure food imaginable. This approach is impractical and unrealistic, because we need a **general** idea of the fat content of different foods. It's not helpful to know the amount of cholesterol in llama tongues or sheep brains. Another strategy is to stick to one healthy food and beat it to death. There are stores stuffed with low fat cookbooks extolling the virtues of soya bean salad, soya bean quiche, and soya bean pancakes. These reference works are probably too specific for those who need to understand the difference between olive oil and motor oil (olive oil is better with fish).

Scientifically based dietary advice is the central component of a cholesterol-lowering program. Spending just a few hours learning about nutrition can fulfill your goal of reducing your cholesterol. Contrary to the beliefs of many, not all fats have negative effects on health. Fat is a vital component of our diet. It is imperative to understand that there are different types of fat, both good and bad.

Learning to read packages is very important. Companies will often do whatever they can to champion the nutritional benefits of their product while hiding or misrepresenting the ingredients that are harmful. As a result, packaging can be extremely sly and deceptive. Understanding a few basic rules about food labels is essential. Because most of us are more attracted to the colour of the package than its contents, encouraging people to read and understand unintelligible small print can be a challenge.

Various types of dietary fats are listed in table 6. After a brief discourse on these, you will learn about smart dietary decisions based on the fat content of various foods. This will be complemented by an explanation of the confusing jargon which often occupies the entire label of processed foods.

Table 6

DIETARY FATS

1. Cholesterol
2. Saturated fat
3. Unsaturated fat
   — monounsaturated fat
   — polyunsaturated fat

4. Modified vegetable oils (saturated)
   — hydrogenated vegetable oil
   — partially hydrogenated vegetable oil
   — transfatty acids

Cholesterol

Cholesterol is the most recognized fat and the easiest to understand. There is no such thing as good or bad dietary cholesterol. For cardiac patients, it is all bad. Though some is essential, especially in children, Western diets include far too much. Only about 10% of the calories in our diet should be in the form of cholesterol. Many people eat three or four times this recommendation.

Though it is commonly understood that cholesterol avoidance is important, the rationale remains vague to most of us. To capitalize on name recognition, there are a multitude of products which trumpet themselves as cholesterol-free. Unbeknownst to many people, **cholesterol is only found in foods of animal origin**, either dairy or meat. Therefore, advertising a bag of potato chips or crackers as cholesterol-free is like saying a sack of carrots contains no onions, or that a cheesecake is "chickenless." This is flagrantly deceptive marketing masquerading as nutritional wisdom. **Cholesterol-free does not mean fat-free.** Many products contain no cholesterol (some taco chips, cookies, cakes, and pies) but still have enormous amounts of other unhealthy fats lurking in the shadows, waiting to take up residence in the walls of your coronary arteries.

The cholesterol in your blood comes from two sources: it is absorbed from your diet and manufactured by your liver. There is no saturation mechanism for the intestinal absorption of cholesterol, so the more you eat, the higher your blood cholesterol will be. About half of the cholesterol we eat is absorbed and the rest passes through the intestines as waste. Blood levels increase by an average of 15% on a high cholesterol diet. There are wide variations in individual responses because of various factors like genetics. Dietary cholesterol accounts for only some of the cholesterol transported by lipoproteins (LDL and HDL), since the liver produces so much. Therefore, if you were to embark on a zero-cholesterol diet, cholesterol made by the liver would still circulate in your body.

There is an important difference between dietary cholesterol and blood cholesterol. This is because blood levels are influenced by more than simply dietary intake. **Cholesterol will change in response to the ingestion of *all* dietary fats.** In other words, if you lower your cholesterol intake but still pig out on other high fat foods, your blood cholesterol will remain elevated or rise. I have seen scores of patients frustrated by the lack of any real progress in their cholesterol despite cutting out most of their dietary intake. The problem is that they are still eating enough fat from other sources to heat their homes for a year. In order to have a tangible effect on the lipid profile, cholesterol intake must be altered as part of a larger dietary program to reduce total fat, particularly the saturated kind.

Dietary Fats

The ensuing discussion may be a bit more detailed than expected. Though I endeavour to simplify it to the barest essentials, you may still pass out.

Cholesterol is one important dietary fat, but there are others. They are **saturated** fats (bad) and **unsaturated** fats (good). Unsaturated fats are further classified as either **monounsaturated** or **polyunsaturated**. Saturated and unsaturated fats are constructed of **fatty acids.** Fatty acids look like long necklaces. When three of them get together, they form a **triglyceride**. The type of fatty acid that makes up the triglyceride determines whether we are eating heart-attack-provoking **saturated fats** or healthy **unsaturated fats**. Most of our dietary fat is in the form of triglycerides or cholesterol.

Saturated fats are unhealthy because they raise cholesterol. Therefore, both dietary cholesterol and dietary saturated fat increase your risk of having a heart attack. Unsaturated fats have a more innocuous and indeterminate effect on blood cholesterol levels and are considered neutral.

Research suggests that **dietary saturated fat has an even greater effect on raising cholesterol than dietary cholesterol does**. Knowing the enemy is the key to winning the battle, even when the preferred strategy is avoidance. Most people do not understand how to avoid unhealthy fats because they do not know where they are hiding. So let's spend the rest of the chapter tracking down the enemy.

Foods with a high content of saturated fats include cream, butter, cheese, milk, tropical oils, and beef and pork fat such as lard, tallow, and shortening (table 7). Examples of tropical oils are palm oil, palm kernel oil, coconut oil, and cocoa butter. When you see any of these listed on the package, retreat!

Table 7

SOURCES OF SATURATED FAT

1. Beef
2. Bacon
3. Lard
4. Tallow
5. Shortening
6. Cream
7. Butter
8. Cheese
9. Tropical oils
    — palm oil
    — palm kernel oil
    — coconut oil
    — cocoa butter

Hydrogenation

We are not done yet. There are a few other concepts needed to better understand dietary fat. Saturated fat is a complex villain. Though it is present in some foods naturally, it may also be produced by chemically altering unsaturated fats during industrial food processing. Because the result is not listed as "saturated" on food packaging, it is more difficult to recognize the danger. The resulting fats are extremely "atherogenic," meaning they cause narrowing in coronary arteries. The important fat catchwords are listed as **hydrogenated** and **partially hydrogenated vegetable oils** and **transfatty acids**. Most people think vegetable oil is healthy. When it is hydrogenated vegetable oil, though, you might as well inject it directly into your coronaries. Federal regulations do not require transfatty acids to be listed separately on packaging. They are lumped together with the hydrogenated and partially hydrogenated vegetable oils, which should always be looked for on the ingredient list.

Hydrogenation is a chemical transformation in food processing which changes healthy unsaturated fat into unhealthy hydrogenated or partially hydrogenated vegetable oils and transfatty acids. Why bother transforming healthy fat into unhealthy fat when making packaged foods? This process is necessary because unsaturated fats are not naturally shelf-friendly. They are more liquid than solid. This makes them more difficult to integrate into foods. Unsaturated fats are also less palatable, more perishable, and become rancid quickly. They are thus chemically altered and solidified to produce a marketable product with a long shelf life. Someone may have tried marketing liquid crackers once but it didn't take off. (What would you eat them with?) Without hydrogenation to make these fats more solid, you would be purchasing mushy potato chips, runny biscuits, and watery doughnuts. To add one more piece to the dietary puzzle, saturated fats result from complete hydrogenation of vegetable oils, and transfatty acids are produced from partial hydrogenation of vegetable oils.

There are two nutritional considerations with fat: the amount of calories and therefore the risk of adding weight to your lean machine, and their association with raised cholesterol and therefore heart attacks. As we have touched upon, dietary cholesterol raises blood cholesterol and LDL levels. Transfatty acids and hydrogenated and partially hydrogenated vegetable oils do the same. In addition, transfatty acids lower HDL (the good stuff) and have been linked to an increased risk of breast cancer.

You now have a framework from which to modify your diet. I have explained what cholesterol, saturated fats, hydrogenation, and transfatty acids are. The last fats to talk about are **unsaturated**, which can be either polyunsaturated or monounsaturated. These are the healthier fats. They do not have the same negative effects on coronary arteries as the others. When you read about fish being a healthy choice, this is partly due to its high content of unsaturated fats. One reason Inuit and Japanese have such a low incidence of coronary disease is their taste for fish, and their limited intake of more unhealthy fats.

Monounsaturated Fats

Fats are classified according to their different chemical structures and, without drowning you in details, monounsaturated fats have a different chemical structure than saturated fats. This has an impact on the way they are used by the body, hence their **atherogenicity**, or propensity to cause coronary artery disease. Monounsaturated fats, present in oils like sunflower, canola (rapeseed), olive, and safflower, do not raise blood cholesterol levels (table 8). Pistachios, avocados, and salmon are rich sources of monounsaturates. Oils high in monounsaturated fat may actually **lower** cholesterol. This probably relates to the replacement of dietary saturated fat with monounsaturated fats when eating habits change. Though monounsaturated fats probably do not have a direct effect on lowering cholesterol, there is no evidence that they will raise them either.

Table 8

SOURCES OF MONOUNSATURATED FAT

1. Sunflower oil
2. Safflower oil
3. Canola oil
4. Olive oil
5. Pistachios
6. Avocados
7. Salmon
8. Mackerel

Polyunsaturated Fats

This is the final fat. Polyunsaturated fatty acids, or PUFA, are known as the "essential" fatty acids. They merit this title because they are integral to our daily functioning. Whereas cholesterol is manufactured by the liver and the other fats are not a requisite part of our diet, we are incapable of producing PUFA. They are synthesized by plants. PUFA have a variety of indispensable metabolic roles.

We could not survive without them. A body without PUFA is like a car without oil; eventually, it would wear out and no longer function. The two important types of PUFA are **omega-3** and **omega-6**. The names seem more appropriate for space exploration and are probably part of a scientific conspiracy to confuse the populace. They have been linked with various beneficial effects, including a reduced incidence of coronary disease and fewer sudden cardiac deaths. These fats are predominantly found in fish oils (and therefore fish). PUFA are also found in vegetable oils such as safflower, corn, soy, canola, and sunflower.

A heart attack occurs when a complete obstruction in a coronary artery obstructs flow. This happens when a blood clot develops over a lipid-filled narrowing. This explains why aspirin is an effective medication in heart disease. Aspirin keeps blood thin, which inhibits clotting and therefore prevents heart attacks. PUFA also have anti-clotting ability, which may explain the association of a high PUFA diet with a reduction in sudden cardiac death. Another benefit is a favourable effect on blood cholesterol. While a high PUFA diet has been shown to lower LDL, there is also evidence HDL is lowered. The practical importance of these inconsistent findings is unclear, though diets high in PUFA have been associated with a **reduction** in coronary artery disease.

So now we know that dietary fat includes cholesterol, saturated fats (including hydrogenated and partially hydrogenated vegetable oils and transfatty acids), monounsaturated fats, and polyunsaturated fats. Cholesterol is exclusively of animal origin while the others may be found in plants or animals.

Dietary Advice

Nutrition experts are paid piles of money by governments to ascertain the proper combination of nutrients in a healthy diet. Based on scientific studies, panels of specialists recommend the precise mix of fat, protein, carbohydrates, vitamins, and minerals needed to maintain optimal health. There is even a separate menu for those with heart disease. Though such recommendations are important as **guidelines**, it is unreasonable to expect people to dash to grocery stores with calculators and weigh scales to compute the exact amount of cholesterol and transfatty acids in their shopping carts. I think it is better to paint the canvas with broader strokes.

Though I will provide some detailed information, my purpose is to provide specifics from which you can intelligently generalize. For example, I can tell you how much cholesterol there is in a two-ounce shrimp, but I think you would be quickly ostracized from your social circles if you took this too literally. ("Sure, I'd love a Cajun shrimp — how much does it weigh?") The important information is that shrimps are very high in cholesterol. This is not intended to condemn you to a shrimpless existence, but moderation is important. The definition of moderation is up to you and I can only provide guidelines for common sense. A low fat diet is common sense. It should be dominated by fruits, vegetables, grains, beans, and pastas. It is easy to regulate fat intake once you learn which foods to avoid. A high fat or high cholesterol treat should be no more than a weekly occurrence, and even then, only if you must.

I occasionally hear the argument that food is so important to some people, a life devoid of creamy rich dessert is not worth living. I have two responses to this. Firstly, priorities should be clearly and firmly set. If food is that central to a patient's life, then this priority needs to be modified or there is little reason to expect dietary habits to change. An awareness of risk implies an acceptance of risk. Motivation has to exist before changes can be made. I acknowledge that this oversimplifies an extremely complex issue, but dietary advice is not intended for hardened food addicts. Most people should be capable of altering bad eating habits without requiring psychotherapy and acupuncture. The second response to this argument is that there is a dizzying array of tasty low fat choices for heart-healthy diets. Some people believe such a diet is so insipid and tasteless that they would rather die young eating bacon and eggs than live to 100 on tofu and broccoli. That is freedom of choice. I maintain that it simply requires a little time and effort to find choices suitable for your tastebuds and healthy for your heart.

A Mathematical Digression

Dietary recommendations are quantified by calories and depend on body weight and activity level. A **calorie** is a measure of energy which is required by all people at all times. Weightlifters require more calories than pencil pushers (unless it is an extremely heavy pencil). The more calories consumed, the more must be expended to prevent their storage as fat (i.e., spare tires). Fat is associated with weight gain because it contains nine calories per gram, whereas proteins and carbohydrates have only four calories per gram. **Therefore, gram for gram, two and a quarter more calories are eaten on a high fat diet than a high carbohydrate diet.** Reread those last two sentences. Very simple yet profoundly important information. The average fat content in Western diets is 40% of ingested calories. This number should always be less than 30%, and less than 15–20% for those with coronary artery disease or coronary risk factors. Mediterranean-style diets, which include lots of pasta, beans, and vegetables are about 15% fat. The most important points about fat are the amount and type consumed.

Table 9

RECOMMENDED DAILY FAT INTAKE

Calories	Total Fat (grams)				
	10%	15%	20%	25%	30%
1,200	13	20	27	33	40
1,400	15	23	31	39	47
1,600	18	27	36	44	53
1,800	20	30	40	50	60
2,000	22	33	44	56	67
2,200	24	37	49	61	73
2,400	26	40	54	67	80
2,600	29	43	58	72	87
2,800	31	47	62	78	93
3,000	33	50	67	83	100

Use this table in conjunction with information about the fat content of foods to learn exactly how much fat you are eating. Your calorie requirements depend on your activity level and body size. To work out how many calories you need to maintain your body weight, multiply your weight in pounds by 14. For example, a person weighing 165 pounds would need to eat about 2,300 calories.

If you eat 1,500 calories of food and 30% is fat, this is 450 calories of fat (30% of 1,500 is 450). If there are nine calories in one gram of fat, then 450 calories equals 50 grams of fat (450 divided by nine is 50). If 20% of your 1,500 calories was fat, this would be about 33 grams. If Johnny has six cheeseburgers and gives Sally three, what do you have? Two overweight people with heart disease. I recommend all patients give themselves a **fat allowance** in grams based on age, sex, and activity level. See table 9 to determine your fat allowance. Fat content is listed on packaging in grams or milligrams. One gram equals 1,000 mg (milligrams). When you realize how many grams of fat are safe to consume per day, reading food labels will be more helpful in planning your diet.

Cholesterol-Rich Foods

For adults with heart disease or coronary risk factors, the less cholesterol in the diet, the better. The recommended daily intake for cardiac patients is less than 200 mg. There is evidence that diets with an exceptionally sparse fat composition may halt or even reverse coronary disease. Though some extremists advocate this zero-tolerance approach, it is impractical for most people. Some patients may graduate to this level, but initial goals should be more attainable.

Table 10

CHOLESTEROL & FAT CONTENT OF MEATS & SHELLFISH (3-ounce portions)

Meat	Total Fat (g)	Cholesterol (mg)
Mussels	3.9	48
Lobster	0.5	61
Oysters	2.4	52
Scallops	3.3	34
Shrimp	4.5	156
Crab	1.4	45–85
Beef	8.7	77
Lamb	6.8	78
Pork	11.1	79
Veal	4.7	129
Liver	4.0	270
Brain	10.7	1,746
Chicken (light meat)	3.8	72
Chicken (dark meat)	8.2	79
Turkey (light meat)	1.3	59
Turkey (dark meat)	6.1	72

The amount of cholesterol in meat depends on which animal, what part of the animal, and how much of it is consumed. The only way to quantify the cholesterol content of a certain food is to use a **specified weight**. For example, a 3-ounce piece of skinless chicken breast contains about

70 mg of cholesterol. Of course, few people can stop at a mere three ounces at the dinner table. This is a ploy often used as a means to mislead the public. "Only 10 grams of fat per serving," the package will trumpet. When you read the fine print, it is apparent that the "serving" size would not satisfy your pet gerbil (which, incidentally, is low in cholesterol in bite-sized portions). Therefore, the benefit of knowing the cholesterol or fat content of a food depends on adequate knowledge of serving sizes. With that in mind, table 10 should give you an idea of the total fat and cholesterol content of various animal products. Remember that cholesterol is not the only villain. Foods usually contain other fats, both good and bad.

Dietary Oils

Oils are fats with a lower melting temperature. They are liquid at room temperature and contain mostly polyunsaturated and monounsaturated fats. Fats are solid at room temperature, and thus predominantly saturated. Oils and fats are added to most processed foods. They alter our perception of the food we eat by changing its texture. Food texture is very important to many people. It is more enjoyable to eat a food that easily slides into the stomach than one that feels like sandpaper. This is why sand is less popular than mustard and mayonnaise. Fat, in the form of butter, cream, shortening, etc., gives foods its palatability and uniformity. The general population worships fatty food because of its smoothness and richness. Most people would prefer a doughnut, even a celery-flavoured doughnut, to real celery. We devour high fat items not because of a secret desire to be overweight, but because, by their very nature, they satisfy our pleasure centres.

Figure 8 lists common commercially available oils and the amount of fat present in each. No oil contains purely one type of fat. They all have variable amounts of saturated and

Fatty Acid Content of Dietary Fats

(Normalized to 100%)

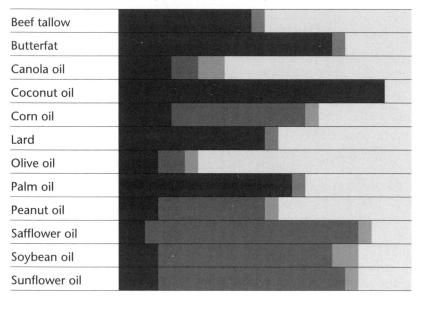

Beef tallow
Butterfat
Canola oil
Coconut oil
Corn oil
Lard
Olive oil
Palm oil
Peanut oil
Safflower oil
Soybean oil
Sunflower oil

Saturated fat   Monounsaturated fat

Polyunsaturated fat (omega-6)

Polyunsaturated fat (omega-3)

FIGURE 8

unsaturated fat. The percentage of these fats determines if the oil is healthy or unhealthy. Whether good or bad, oils still contain plenty of calories to overinsulate your frame. When any oil is heated above 185 degrees Celsius for more than 15 minutes, **it is converted to the hydrogenated form** and rendered atherogenic (i.e., unhealthy).

If an oil sounds as if you are taking a vacation then it is bad for you. This includes the tropical oils such as palm oil, palm kernel oil, and coconut oil. They are saturated and therefore raise blood cholesterol. They are present in many packaged foods and are the main fat in chocolates. If you must indulge in these on vacation, smear them on your skin. On packaging, ingredients are listed in a way to dupe you into a sense of false security. An explanation of the ingredient is not required. Though coconut oil may not have meant anything to you before, you now know to be wary of it. Other common dietary fats are lard, tallow, and butterfat. Once again these are sources of large amounts of saturated fat, and foods with these listed on their packages should be eschewed by the heart-healthy patient and banished from the cupboards. Cookies and potato chips are simply unacceptable snacks for patients worried about coronary artery disease. Pick up an apple or carrot at the market instead.

The sources of vegetable oils are varied. They are extracted from nuts, seeds, or part of the grain called germ (e.g., corn oil). The healthiest oils are canola, safflower, sunflower, and corn. These are preferable choices for cooking since they contain much more unsaturated fat (polyunsaturated and monounsaturated) than saturated fat. But remember that cooking at high temperatures for too long will turn unsaturated to saturated fat, making your meal unhealthy.

Poultry

Skinless chicken and turkey are usually lower in cholesterol and fat than other meat sources such as beef, pork, lamb, and veal. Light meat has marginally less cholesterol and **much less total fat** than its darker counterpart. **Duck** has more fat than either chicken or turkey, especially domestic as opposed to wild duck. This makes it one of the less desirable members of the poultry family for a heart-healthy diet. Birds should never be eaten with skin (or feathers) by those interested in lowering cholesterol and reducing weight. In its role as an insulator, skin contains enormous amounts of fat and cholesterol. Cooking poultry with the skin attached is equally bad since the fatty drippings are absorbed into the meat. As for **chicken wings**, there is so little meat on those teeny things, if you remove the skin you end up with nothing but a few bones. Avoid them.

Brains & Other Bits

When travelling through Turkey, I was surprised to see sheep's brain salad offered in restaurants. **Brain** has more cholesterol than any other body part by far. A three-ounce portion of brain has 20 times the cholesterol content as the same amount of beef. However, zombie movies aside, brain has yet to take off in the North American fast food market and I do not foresee a chain of "Mr. Brains" doing brisk business in the near future.

Another dietary hazard of eating brains is **kuru,** a degenerative brain disease. An obscure tribe in New Guinea honour their deceased relatives by mixing their brains (the relatives' brains, that is) in a gourd of ashes and drinking it. The problem is that many of the brains harbour organisms called prions, the cause of kuru. This ritual cannibalistic practice results in transmission of the prion from generation to generation in the brain tissue of affected relatives. The lesson is that if you have a choice between eating your deceased relative or erecting a tombstone, choose the latter.

Though the cholesterol content of **liver** does not approach that of brain, it remains a rich source of this villainous fat. This makes sense since the liver is the mammalian manufacturing centre of cholesterol. Popular patés of duck and beef are mostly liver. Try a tofu spread instead. Ox testicle soup is a popular Middle Eastern delicacy. I don't know how much cholesterol such soup contains and I have no plans to research it.

Red Meat

Though **veal** contains about 60% more cholesterol than beef, lamb, and pork, it has nearly half the total fat content.

Of the four meats, **pork** has more total fat than all of the others. Red meat should always be purchased as lean as possible. **Prime grade** hamburger contains up to 40% fat. After cooking a three-and-a-half-ounce hamburger you are left with about 100 grams. If 40% of this is fat, then you are consuming 40 grams of fat, about 20 of which are saturated. If you represent the typical person and eat 2,000 calories a day, then you should only be consuming about 20 grams of saturated fat daily. Accordingly, one prime grade burger essentially blows the wad. **Choice grade** is the more usual store-purchased hamburger and has about 20–25% fat, which amounts to 12–15 grams of saturated fat. **Choice grade–diet lean** hamburger has 15–20% fat, and **select beef**, 10%. If you have to satisfy your carnivorous instincts (and tastebuds), go for the leanest meat. The downside is the extra expense of low fat meat. If you really need meat but can't stand the thought of feasting on high fat offerings, buffalo is a low-fat beef alternative. Impractical unless you're one of the Flintstones, but low fat.

More Red Meat

There are numerous ways of limiting the fat content of a beef meal. Some parts of the animal are less fatty than others. **Select** cuts have less fat than **choice** cuts (table 11). **Round** steaks generally have the least saturated fat and cholesterol, though they may be less tasty. **Loins** (such as sirloin and tenderloin) are very unhealthy. A 10-ounce slab of beef tenderloin has 40 grams of fat, compared to an eye of round steak which has under 10 grams. A 10-ounce porterhouse has over 60 grams of fat and a similar portion of untrimmed beef short ribs contain enough fat to fill all your coronary arteries and those of your spouse — over 120 grams. So when you decide to eat a steak, you might as well choose the best of the worst. All visible fat should be trimmed before cooking or it will be absorbed into the meat.

In addition, fat content is affected by the method of cooking. Putting meat on the BBQ or broiling it will remove some fat. This is far superior to frying meat, which allows it to bathe in fat and oil. Processed meats, like bologna, salami, and sausages, are extremely unhealthy choices (right up there with chicken wings and ribs). They are very high in fat and should be completely (yes, completely) avoided.

Table 11

BEEF
(10 ounce portions)

Higher Fat *(content in grams)*	Lower Fat *(content in grams)*
Choice cuts	*Select cuts*
1. Short ribs — 115	1. Eye of round — 12
2. Chuck blade roast — 70	2. Top round — 15
3. Chuck arm pot roast — 70	3. Bottom round — 17
4. Porterhouse steak — 60	4. Tip round — 20
5. Top sirloin (choice) — 45	5. Top sirloin (select) — 20
6. Top loin — 35	
7. Beef tenderloin — 40	

Soya

Not sauce, protein. Substituting **soya protein** (this is a vegetable protein source more commonly referred to as tofu) for animal protein reduces cholesterol, LDL, and triglycerides. This effect is greatest in people with the highest lipids who eat the most soya. It is not as meaty a taste as the real thing, but you would have to fill your garage with it to get the same amount of fat present in a sirloin, and soya has no cholesterol or saturated fat. Whereas most vegetable sources of protein are nutritionally incomplete, the protein content of soya is comparable to meat. Just how soya protein affects lipid values has been a subject of great interest. The beneficial effects may be mediated by naturally occurring estrogens in the soya known as **isoflavones**. These estrogens are extremely weak, so men need not worry about developing urges to wear garters and stockings (unless the urges predated the soya ingestion).

Fish

Fish and seafood contain lots of fat. They are distinguished from land-based meat by the type and amount. Whereas beef has plenty of cholesterol and saturated fat, seafood has varying amounts of cholesterol and little saturated fat. Fish contains large amounts of healthy monounsaturated and polyunsaturated fats. Table 12 lists the fat composition of different seafood items.

Shellfish such as shrimps, lobsters, crabs, and clams are high in cholesterol and low in saturated fat. Three-ounce **shrimps** have lots of cholesterol (about 160 mg) while the same amount of **scallops** have little (about 35 mg). **Lobster** has about 60 mg of cholesterol in a three-ounce serving, which is probably as much as most people can afford anyway. Interestingly, lobster has scarce amounts of saturated and unsaturated fats. Based on cholesterol content alone, shrimp and lobster should be reserved for special occasions. **Tuna** has less cholesterol and fat than **salmon**, and both have less than shellfish. Of course, this depends on the serving size. A 10-pound tuna sandwich definitely has more cholesterol than a puny two-ounce shrimp. Therefore, this information presumes comparable portions.

Populations with high fish diets, such as Inuit in Greenland, have among the lowest rates of coronary disease in the world. Most North Americans are ill-prepared for a life in Greenland. We prefer to buy seal meat in the frozen food section of the grocery, and not in a kiosk on an ice floe from a fisherman with a harpoon in his hand. Thankfully, the culinary habits of the Inuit can be copied without learning to hunt sea lions and narwhals. Simply eat more fish.

What do we know about the cardiac effects of high fish diets? Studies have shown everything from a reduction in sudden cardiac death from eating one fatty fish meal per week, to fewer extra heartbeats in people who take 15 ml of cod liver oil. Patients who have had a heart attack live longer on a high fish diet, defined as at least two portions of "fatty fish" per week (i.e., salmon, tuna, herring, mackerel, halibut, etc.). Leaner fish include cod, sole, and haddock. In another study which looked at the fish-eating habits of men over a 30-year period, two portions of fish per week was shown to protect against fatal heart attacks. What remains unclear is whether the fish oil (the polyunsaturated fat called omega-3), or perhaps some other part of the fish (gills or scales perhaps?), is responsible for the benefit. Regardless, a diet rich in fish will reduce your heart attack risk.

Table 12

FAT CONTENT OF FISH
grams of fat per 3 ounces, either baked, broiled, or steamed

	CALORIES	TOTAL FAT	MONO. FAT	POLY. FAT	OMEGA-3	OMEGA-6	SAT. FAT	CHOLEST. (mg)
Herring*	220	12.5	5	3	2.3	0.25	2.8	83
Cod	90	0.8	0.1	0.3	0.1	0.03	0.1	47
Haddock	95	0.8	0.1	0.2	0.2	0.04	0.1	63
Sole	100	1.3	0.3	0.4	0.5	0.05	0.3	58
Trout	129	5.0	1.4	1.5	1.0	0.35	1.4	59
Salmon	185	9.4	4.5	2.1	1.1	0.12	1.6	74
Mackerel	221	15.2	5.9	3.7	1.1	0.16	3.5	64
Tuna	156	5.4	1.7	1.5	1.2	0.10	1.4	42
Sardines**	180	9.9	3.3	4.4	1.2	3.04	1.3	122

* smoked ** in oil, drained

It is important to remember that those who reside in the Arctic traditionally eat a whole heck of a lot of fish and do a lot of physical activity to get it. As a result, their incidence of heart disease is very low for this combination of reasons. But, pound for pound, fish is healthier than meat, and I advocate that all cardiac patients eat a minimum of two portions per week.

À La Carte

This synopsis describes meat "à la carte," but no one eats it without sauce or flavouring. This is an easy way to make an otherwise healthy meal unhealthy. Frying your catch of the day in batter, smothering it in a creamy béarnaise sauce, or dipping it in melted butter are a few ways to negate the beneficial effects. Alfredo sauces are a white creamy death. Many of us attempt to rationalize our poor eating habits. We assuage our guilt with a diet cola to accompany buttered popcorn and cheese nachos. A salad will not negate the atherogenic effects of a hamburger, fries, and cheesecake. The salad is a lone voice in a sea of lard, and it will be swallowed up.

Fast Food

Fast food is synonymous with convenience and the faster it is the more convenient it is. Despite the popularity of these outlets, you have to diligently search the menu to find nutritious options. Grilled offerings are better than fried ones. Forget mayo, cheese, and creamy dressings. Fast food chicken sandwiches are healthier than burgers, as table 13 illustrates.

It is not only the beef patty which makes nutritionists shriek in horror at the words Big Mac. The addition of cheese and ranch dressing make a Big Mac an extremely unhealthy choice for lunch. It is 55% fat by weight. It should be called Fat Mac or Big Fat or Big Fat Mac. I believe in moderation, however, and every so often, maybe once a year, I will **think** of eating one. Table 14 lists the fat content of one popular fast food outlet.

Table 13

FAST FOOD COMPARISON

	Total fat (g)	Sat. fat (g)	Calories
Harvey's			
Grilled Chicken Supreme	5	1	300
McDonald's			
Grilled Chicken Deluxe	6	1	330
Wendy's			
Big Bacon Classic	30	12	580
Burger King			
Whopper with Cheese	46	16	730

Table 14

FAST FOOD FAT

	Calories	Fat Percentage
Big Mac	500	45% (26 g)
Egg McMuffin	300	40% (14 g)
Quarter Pounder & Cheese	535	50% (30 g)
Quarter Pounder	425	45% (21 g)
McChicken	500	45% (24 g)
Small Fries	250	40% (12 g)
Filet-O-Fish	350	40% (15 g)
Chicken McNuggets (6)	230	45% (12 g)
House Dressing (pkg.)	200	95% (21 g)
Sausage McMuffin & Egg	500	60% (32 g)
Scrambled Eggs	160	55% (11 g)
Hot Mustard Sauce	65	50% (3.5 g)

Though this provides a sample of a typical McDonald's menu, Wendy's, Harvey's, Burger King, Kentucky Fried Chicken, and many other fast food outlets are similar.

Butter & Margarine

Smooth creamy butter goes well with many things, including caskets and tombstones. It is the paragon of saturated fats and is loaded with them. Butter is used in processed foods because it enriches taste and texture. One five-gram pat of butter contains about four grams of fat, two-thirds of which is saturated. Butter approaches bacon on the health food scale, meaning it isn't even on the scale. Low fat butter still contains 40% fat. Buttering bread is unnecessary. Dip it in your soup, dip it in your water, dip it on the floor, but don't dip it in butter. Margarine, though no golden angel, is better than butter. This is apparent by examining their respective consistencies. Butter, being solid, is composed of saturated fats. Because margarine is softer, it has less saturated fat and thus less potential to raise cholesterol and obstruct coronary arteries, presuming it is low in transfatty acids.

A recent study showed that patients who chose margarine in their diet had lower cholesterol readings than those eating butter. Not all margarines are created equal. In some, hydrogenated vegetable oils and transfatty acids predominate. This is apparent from the ingredient list. Look to see if hydrogenated vegetable oil is listed first or near the top. They are much more unhealthy than the lower fat alternatives and should be ridiculed, dodged, ostracized, and perhaps stoned. Examples of acceptable margarines are listed in table 15.

Table 15

MARGARINES — *Acceptable brands**

Becel Salt Free
Becel Light
Becel Non-Hydrogenated
Fleischmann's Tub Sunflower Oil
Fleischmann's Tub Corn Oil
Fleischmann's Low Sodium
Fleischmann's Non-Hydrogenated
I Can't Believe It's Not Butter
Blue Bonnet
Country Crock
Lactantia Unsalted
Lactantia Olivina Non-Hydrogenated
Too Good To Be True

*Read the package to make sure that hydrogenated oil is not the first ingredient.

Garlic

Garlic is well-known for its anti-vampire capabilities. It has also been touted as a remedy for high cholesterol. Truth or fiction? This depends on whether you manufacture the stuff. Early studies suggested that garlic was capable of **minimally** reducing blood cholesterol (perhaps enough to extend your life by four hours). The methods of these studies were poor. In a more recent and rigorous trial, no beneficial effects were demonstrated. If your primary goals are to spice up your food and spice down your love life, then use garlic with reckless abandon. If you think it will reduce your cholesterol, recent evidence suggests you are wasting your money.

Eggs

Because I have not alienated enough farmers, it is worth saying a few words about eggs (table 16). The unfortunate characteristic of eggs is their naturally indivisible nature, which is the egg white and the egg yolk. There is no disputing the nutritional benefit of eggs. If my airplane crashed in the Andes, I would pack soccer balls for recreation and eggs for sustenance. But it is equally indisputable that egg yolks are a source of large amounts of cholesterol, about 200-300 mg per egg. **This approximates the entire daily allowance for a cardiac patient on a low fat diet**. Though special interest groups will continue to market eggs as part of a healthy lifestyle, I believe that eggs should be placed in the same category as bacon, butter, and béarnaise sauce. A number of years ago, a reputable medical journal reported an elderly man who ate dozens of eggs a day for most of his life. He had no evidence of coronary artery disease and a normal lipid profile. This is an exception and not the rule. The more eggs you eat, the higher your risk of heart disease.

Table 16

EGGS
(large hard or soft boiled of 50 grams)

1. Total fat — 5.3 g
2. Cholesterol — 213 mg
3. Saturated fat — 1.6 g
4. Monounsaturated fat — 2.0 g
5. Polyunsaturated fat — 0.7 g
6. Protein — 6.3 g
7. Carbohydrates 0.6 g
8. Sodium — 62 mg
9. Potassium — 62 mg

Cheese & Milk

Dairy products can be very high in cholesterol and saturated fat (table 17). The fat content of these items is listed as a percentage of milk fat (M.F.) or butter fat (B.F.) by weight. If a package of cheese says 30% M.F., then there are 30 grams of fat for every 100 grams of cheese. This is *way* too much fat. **Most cheeses list the percentage of milk fat they contain.** The results will surprise you since many are 30% or 40% M.F. Regular cheeses are too high in fat to be safely consumed on a regular basis. A serving of cream cheese has about the same amount of fat as a similar serving of cheddar cheese. Forget the cheese and choose a piece of fruit. Cheeses produced with skim or partially skim milk are available. If you can't live without your cheese, they are acceptable **alternatives**, but still contain 10–15% fat.

Table 17

CHOLESTEROL & FAT CONTENT OF CHEESE

	Size (g)	Fat (g)	Cholesterol (mg)
Regular fat cheddar	60	18	60
Reduced fat (~15% M.F.)	60	9	30
Low fat (% M.F. [Milk Fat])	60	4	20

Milk is available as whole, 2% fat, 1% fat, or skim (table 18). Understanding the effect of fat on the palate is easy when you compare the taste and texture of different milks. Cream has 10-20% fat. Whole milk has roughly twice as much total fat as 2%, which in turn has twice as much as 1% milk. I find it hard to discern much of a difference between 2% and 1% so I drink the latter. Cardiac patients with concerns about their lipid levels should stick to 1% or skim. Skim may be a problem because it tastes like wet paper, although it's all in what you're used to.

As with all dietary selections, milk, cheese, or yogurt should be chosen according to the fat content listed on the package. Ice cream is very high in fat and calories. There are a variety of fat-free ices and sherbets on the market which are equally fulfilling to a sweet tooth (except the garlic-flavoured ones).

Table 18

CHOLESTEROL & FAT CONTENT OF MILK

	Amount (ml)	Fat (g)	Cholesterol (mg)
Whole	500	18	70
2%	500	10	40
1%	500	5	20
Skim	500	1	10

Packaging

It is worth reiterating that cholesterol-free does not mean fat-free. Don't be fooled. When a product has "light" listed on the label, this does not necessarily mean light in fat. It could mean light taste, texture, or even colour. You should never make assumptions about packages. They are designed to entice you to buy the product, not to educate you. When a product has "light" on the package, it must specify what part of the product is light. Perhaps it's the packaging itself which is light.

When a package makes a claim about a specific fat — for example, "low in cholesterol" — then a list of all fat contained in that product is mandatory. As a result, you will be able to see the exact amounts of cholesterol, saturated, monounsaturated, and polyunsaturated fat it contains. The list may refer to a serving size different from that listed on the package. For example, a 100-gram bag of taco chips may list the fat content of a 50-gram serving, so always compare serving size and package size. You may be consuming more fat than you think.

Table 19

PACKAGING RULES

1. "Fat Free" — less than 0.1 grams of fat per 100-gram serving
2. "Low Fat" — less than 3 grams of fat per serving
3. "100% Vegetable Oil" — no cholesterol, but may be full of hydrogenated vegetable oil or transfatty acids.
4. "Cholesterol Free" — less than 3 mg of cholesterol per 100 grams or per serving.
5. "Low Cholesterol" — less than 20 mg of cholesterol per 100 grams or per serving.

Nutrition labelling is voluntary unless a health claim is made, in which case it must be substantiated. Some specific regulations exist in the world of food packaging (table 19). One interesting example is the requirement of a nutritional breakdown if health claims such as "light," "low fat," or "hamster entrails-free" are advertised. One ploy used by those with a special interest in hiding unhealthy ingredients is to list contents in difficult-to-understand terms. Though monopolyglutacarbonifrits is not a household word, if you read it on a package you would probably perceive it as unhealthy (I made it up anyway). There are various ingredients which when translated nutritionally are simply **fat**. These include the transfatty acids and hydrogenated vegetable oils already described. Ingredients are listed on packages in descending order according to the amount present. Therefore, seeing the word "lard" at the top of the list has more serious ramifications than noting it way down at the bottom.

Table 20	
WHAT DO THE PACKAGING CLAIMS REALLY MEAN?	
Package #1	*Package #2*
"cholesterol free"	"cholesterol free"
"low saturates"	"low saturates"
"no tropical oils"	"no tropical oils"
"100% vegetable oil"	"100% vegetable oil"
Nutritional information	Nutritional information
Fat — **6.4** grams	Fat — **3.2** grams
Polyunsaturates — **0.3** grams	Polyunsaturates — **0.1** grams
Monounsaturates — **2.5** grams	Monounsaturates — **1.3** grams
Saturates — **1.2** grams	Saturates — **0.5** grams
Cholesterol — **0** milligrams	Cholesterol — **0** milligrams

Total Fat – (Saturated fat + PUFA + Monounsaturated fat) = Transfatty acid content

Coffee

A recent study compared the effects of filtered coffee and plunger coffee on the lipid profile. Filtered coffee is theoretically preferable since the filter paper removes certain chemicals. A few of these chemicals, enzymes called **diterpenes**, have been weakly linked to heart disease. The plunger coffees minimally raise cholesterol and LDL, and slightly reduce HDL. At least six cups were slurped in this study, implying that large amounts must be consumed before there is any demonstrable effect. Better to stop eating butter first and worry about your coffee consumption later.

Cappuccinos, caffe lattes and café au lait are all made with milk. Whole, skim, 2%, or 1% are all available — just ask the coffee bartender. Though caffeine is a mild stimulant, it does not significantly affect blood pressure or heart rate in small to moderate doses and has never been linked as a precipitant of angina or heart attacks (table 21).

Table 21

CAFFEINE CONTENT OF SELECTED BEVERAGES (mg)

Pepsi (12 oz.)	37
Coca-Cola (12 oz.)	47
Mountain Dew (12 oz.)	55
Jolt Cola (12 oz.)	72
Tea (8 oz.)	70
Instant coffee (8 oz.)	76
Brewed coffee (8 oz.)	137
Espresso (3 oz.)	180

Conclusion

This chapter embodies the philosophy that a little knowledge can result in phenomenal changes for a motivated and health-conscious person. This does not mean that you have merely acquired a little knowledge. On the contrary: you should now be able to make intelligent decisions about your cardiac health. It would have been simple to quadruple the details in this chapter. Thicker books have been written about information I provide in a few paragraphs, but expanding the text is unnecessary. I am not trying to create a country of nutritional biochemists. (The job market is tight enough.) The aim is to give you clear, concise information.

Your view of food will change significantly with this new knowledge. I cannot promise that you will no longer covet tasty though unhealthy items. But the hot dogs (ground fat and cholesterol masquerading as a wiener), french fries (fried in a deluge of unhealthy oil), and ice cream (cream is a dirty word) can't be consumed again without a little guilt. You are now aware of the alternatives, the foods and ingredients to avoid, and the positive effects your choices will have on your cardiac health. This is not a static process and your motivation will increase with your knowledge. No amount of cajoling by a physician will change eating behaviour. The choices remain yours.

POINTS TO REMEMBER

- **Cholesterol is only found in meat and dairy products, and the more cholesterol you eat the more likely it is you will have a heart attack.**

- **Saturated fat also increases your risk of having a heart attack, while unsaturated fats (mono and poly) may decrease your risk.**

- **"Hydrogenation" is an industrial process that produces unhealthy saturated fat (including hydrogenated and partially hydrogenated vegetable oils and transfatty acids) from healthy unsaturated fat.**

- **Unhealthy saturated fats include lard, tallow, palm oil, palm kernel oil, and coconut oil. Rich sources of healthy unsaturated fats are safflower, sunflower, corn, canola, and olive oils, pistachios, avocados, and fish of all types.**

- **Avoid liver, eggs, cheese, processed meats, butter, and never eat anything with skin attached to it. Eat sherbet instead of ice cream. Check the lists in this chapter for the cholesterol and fat contents of many foods. The size of the portion is as important as the fat it contains.**

- **Broil or BBQ and avoid frying and fried food. Baked potatoes (without butter or sour cream) may not taste as good as french fries, but you'll live longer eating baked potatoes than you will eating fried ones.**

- **Avoid fast food outlets, unless it's to use the restroom.**

- **Read the package, read the package, read the package.**

8

FIBRE &
HEART DISEASE

If we all ate more fibre, the world would be healthier, more regular, and conspicuously smellier. Fibre has an enormous role to play in favourably altering the lipid profile. Unfortunately, most patients don't really know what fibre is or where to find it.

Fibre is the indigestible part of plants. When the word plant is tossed about, people think of trees and tulips. From a nutritional perspective, however, plant is the opposite of animal and includes fruits and vegetables. Bran, wheat, and oat are also of plant origin because they are grown and harvested. They are excellent sources of fibre. Whereas some mammals (e.g., cows) are adept at digesting this stuff, humans are incapable of such a bovine feat.

Fibre is a catch-all term for a mixture of substances with diverse effects on the body. Though classified as soluble and insoluble, this terminology is obsolete and irrelevant. Most foods contain an assortment of different types of fibre in various proportions. It is nearly impossible to find naturally occurring fibre in purely insoluble or soluble form.

Plants are a natural source of various types of fibre. Examples of fibre include guar, pectin, psyllium, cellulose, oat bran, mucilages, lignin, and wheat bran. Discussing them individually is complex and unnecessary. Though it may be useful to recognize these terms as reflecting fibre content, it's more important to gain familiarity with foods high in fibre. This entire book is devoted to the militaristic concept of a "need-to-know basis." If the information won't improve your ability to modify your coronary risk factors, then why occupy valuable brain power? I don't believe there are many people who care what "mucilage" is, or at least I hope not.

The important questions are: How does fibre help, what proof exists about its benefits, and where can it be found? As stated earlier, fibre is the indigestible part of plants. Digesting protein and carbohydrates is critical to using nutrients and involves breaking food down into smaller and more manageable pieces. Humans produce numerous enzymes in the stomach and small intestine which assume this dirty job in the bowels of the bowels. These enzymes convert food into minuscule nutrients which are absorbed into the bloodstream. The nutrients are used to drive the engines of the body. We do not produce our own enzymes to digest fibre. We cannot digest coins or plastic either, but they do not lower cholesterol so I don't advocate adding them to your diet. Fibre is a physiologic untouchable. It aimlessly meanders through the intestines virtually unopposed until it comes out in the end, both figuratively and literally.

We can only digest fibre with inside help. The large intestine (i.e., the colon) is normally home to millions and millions of bacteria. They are usually nonthreatening in a healthy person and merely use the colon as cheap housing. When they see fibre approach from the small intestine, they know their meal has arrived. Some of these bacteria produce their own enzymes to digest fibre in a process called **fermentation.** It results in the production of a few extra nutrients for the body, and millions more bacteria. This extra bacteria increases the weight of stool. Spouses have known for eons that more than just nutrients are produced after a loved one eats a little extra fibre. The process of fermentation releases a voluminous amount of **gas,** including methane, carbon dioxide, and hydrogen. The more fibre you eat, the more gas you produce. The more gas you produce the less likely it is that your colleagues will be happy to see you in the morning. Nonetheless, beans are good for the heart.

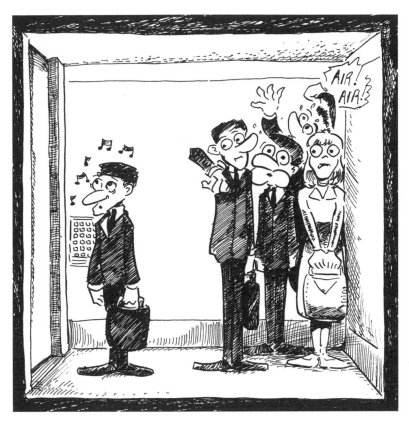

Jerry is on a high fibre diet.

Fibre is a proven and natural therapy for constipation and encourages bowel regularity. Though I expect this is more than you want to know, fibre increases stool volume and makes it less dense by trapping water inside. These larger stools put more pressure on the walls of the bowels and facilitate "passage," a polite term for other *less* polite terms. A high fibre intake must be accompanied by adequate additional fluid or constipation may **increase**. So if you eat more fibre, drink more liquid. Commercial fibre preparations exist in pill and powder form. **Metamucil**, a powdered fibre mixed with water or juice, is an excellent and palatable complement to dietary sources of fibre.

Fibre is responsible for numerous diverse health benefits in addition to bowel regularity. A high fibre diet has been shown to improve blood sugar control in diabetics. These studies have been criticized because participants ingested about 50 grams of fibre, an enormous amount. The benefit of fibre in preventing cancers such as colon cancer is suggestive but has yet to be clearly demonstrated. It may also reduce the risk of breast cancer. One theory is that the fibre binds to cancer-causing agents as they traverse the bowels, kind of like "bowel bouncers." People who switch to a high fibre vegetarian diet have lower blood pressure readings.

What can fibre do to your lipid profile? Many studies have addressed this question. Researchers divided patients into two groups: one group ate a high fibre diet and the other a lower fibre diet. The results are encouraging. High fibre diets can decrease total cholesterol, triglyceride, and LDL by about 20%. HDL may also decrease.

These beneficial effects on lipids occur for two main reasons. The first is known as food displacement. This means that if you eat more fibre you will naturally eat less fat. In this way fibre is not directly lowering cholesterol. Eating a television set would be expected to have the same effect. The second reason is more specific. As fibre courses through the intestine, it actually binds with dietary fat (bowel bouncers again). This reduces fat absorption and results in lower lipid levels.

How much fibre is enough and which foods contain the most? The average North American diet includes about 10 grams of fibre. The recommended intake is 25–30 grams, and some studies have tested two or three times this amount to uncover a positive effect on the lipid profile. Eat more fibre, and you will lower your blood cholesterol and reduce your chances of developing coronary artery disease. The U.S. government is so convinced of this that foods containing enough of it are allowed to trumpet the benefits of fibre on their packages. Table 23 is a list of fibre-rich foods.

Table 22

FIBRE

Benefits	*Adverse effects*

Benefits

1. CONSTIPATION
   promotes bowel regularity and smoothness
2. DIABETES
   improves blood sugar control
3. CANCER
   likely reduces incidence of colon cancer; may reduce incidence of breast cancer
4. BLOOD PRESSURE
   lowers blood pressure
5. LIPID PROFILE
   lowers LDL, triglycerides, and total cholesterol

Adverse effects

1. GAS
   produces more
2. LIPID PROFILE
   lowers HDL (minimally)

Table 23

FIBRE CONTENT OF SELECTED FOOD (grams)

CEREALS (1 oz.)

Fiber One, General Mills	13.0
Kellogg's All-Bran	10.0
Post Raisin Bran	5.9
Post Bran Flakes	5.7
Kellogg's Bran Flakes	5.0
Kellogg's Raisin Bran	5.0
Total Raisin Bran	4.0
Wheat Chex	3.7
Quaker Instant Oatmeal	2.8
Shredded Wheat	2.6
Cheerios	2.0
Kellogg's Corn Flakes	1.0
Froot Loops	1.0
Cap'n Crunch	0.8
Rice Krispies	0
Special K	0

FRUITS

Apple (medium)	3.0
Apricots (three medium)	1.4
Banana (medium)	1.8
Blueberries (one cup)	3.3

Cantaloupe (one cup of pieces) 1.3
Dates (10) 4.2
Figs (10) 7.4
Grapefruit (1/2 medium) 0.7
Kiwi (medium) 2.6
Mango (medium) 2.2
Nectarine (medium) 2.2
Orange (medium) 2.9
Peach (medium) 1.4
Pear (medium) 4.3
Pineapple (one cup of pieces) 1.9
Prunes (10) 6.0
Raisins (2/3 cup) 5.3
Raspberries (1 cup) 5.8
Strawberries (1 cup) 3.9

VEGETABLES (1/2 cup)
Asparagus 1.1
Broccoli 1.2
Brussel sprouts 3.4
Carrot (medium) 2.3
Cauliflower 1.2
Chickpeas 5.7
Corn 3.0
Green beans 1.1
Kidney beans 3.2
Lima beans 6.8
Mushrooms 0.5
Navy beans 3.3
Onions 1.3
Green peas 2.0
Pinto beans 3.4
Sweet peppers 0.8
Potato (medium, no skin) 1.8
Red beans 5.6
Soybean — Miso 7.5
Soybean — Tofu 1.5
Spinach 0.7
Squash 0.8
Sweet potato (medium, with skin) 3.4
Tomato (medium) 1.6
White beans 4.0
Popcorn (3 cups) 2–3

POINTS TO REMEMBER

- Fibre, which comes from plant sources, cannot be digested.

- Drink extra liquid on a high fibre diet or constipation may occur.

- High fibre diets are very healthy and lower cholesterol and LDL.

- Fibre lowers cholesterol by binding to it, thus preventing its absorption.

- Dietary goals are:
  — lose weight if needed
  — reduce cholesterol intake
  — reduce saturated fat intake
  — increase fibre intake

9

VITAMINS & HEART DISEASE

Most patients would prefer to treat their illnesses with "natural" medical remedies. Fear of inadvertent poisoning or hideous side effects is a powerful deterrent from using prescribed "unnatural" synthetic pills. Such fear has spawned a multibillion-dollar supplement industry which I believe puts income and profit above health and welfare. Federal regulations place the burden of disproof on the government. In other words, those peddling herbal supplements do not need to prove a vitamin or herb is safe or effective before marketing it. The government must prove it to be unsafe. As a result, people are shelling out piles of dough on some products which at best do nothing and at worst are harmful. Unfortunately, there are no zero-risk options in medicine, and "natural" should not be mistaken for "risk free."

Vitamin A & Beta-Carotene

Vitamins and herbs are assumed to have mystical healing properties, despite proof that some are categorically dangerous. Many of us simply believe what we want to despite evidence to the contrary. It will be interesting to see the public response to a recent scientific study which examined the benefits of taking **beta-carotene supplements** (a precursor to vitamin A) and **vitamin A** for the prevention of heart disease and cancer. The study was initiated because of

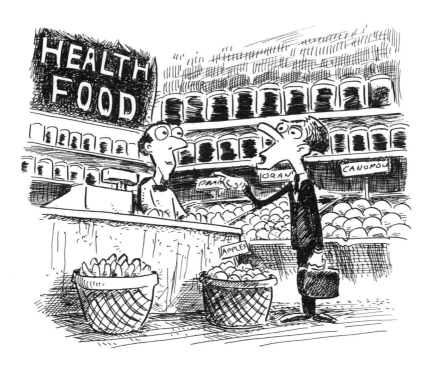

*"Excuse me, I'm looking for vitamin supplements,
but all I see are vegetables."*

observations that people who ate foods rich in these substances had high blood levels of beta-carotene and less
cancer and heart disease. The premise was that "supplements" of these vitamins (i.e., pills) would have the same
beneficial effect.

Unfortunately, the study was prematurely discontinued
because evaluation during the trial showed that the vitamins were actually *killing* people when taken in pill form.
The investigation was undertaken in what is known as a
high risk population. The 18,000 people who were studied
were either smokers or worked with asbestos. Their risk of
being diagnosed with cancer, specifically lung cancer, was
very high. Those individuals taking beta-carotene and vitamin A actually developed **more** lung cancer and had **higher**
death rates. The vitamins had the opposite effect of what

was hoped. Similar findings have occurred with other trials involving beta-carotene supplements.

I doubt that health stores cleared their shelves of the offending compounds or stopped dispensing unsafe or unproven nutritional advice. If they really wish to promote good health, they should have a produce section! I suspect that some people continue to take these particular supplements because the scientific evidence does not support their fixed beliefs. Despite these beliefs, vitamin supplementation clearly has the potential to harm.

In a study of beta-carotene in nonsmokers, there was no difference in cancer or heart disease rates in the beta-carotene versus the placebo group. Beta-carotene supplementation in people already on a diet high in fruits and vegetables may actually *increase* the risk of cancer. All of these trials provide compelling evidence that beta-carotene and vitamin A are at best unhelpful, and at worst harmful. In those looking for a natural therapeutic approach for preventing heart disease, beta-carotene is not recommended.

Antioxidants

Beta-carotene and vitamin A are compounds known as **antioxidants**. Antioxidants are thought to reduce the chances of developing a heart attack. Here's how: when LDL (the bad cholesterol) is **oxidized** it becomes "armed and dangerous," and its ability to clog blood vessels is amplified. Prevent the oxidation and the LDL may be disarmed. There are many other similar compounds and I am certainly open to the possibility that one or more of them will be shown to reduce the chances of developing heart disease or cancer. The potential protective effects of these compounds are part of a much more complex picture. Perhaps their value is in conjunction with the other substances present in fruits and vegetables. Once again, a single herbal pill is no remedy. Eat a carrot or a green leafy vegetable instead.

Vitamin E

Vitamin E, another antioxidant, is an example of a more promising "drug" in the fight against heart disease. Evidence to support its use in the prevention of heart attacks is suggestive, though not complete. Whether vitamin E is best ingested in food or whether it may be just as effective in supplement form is unclear. Though large amounts of beta-carotene are available in fruits and vegetables, smaller amounts of vitamin E are found in a typical North American diet. Foods rich in vitamin E include vegetable oils, sunflower seeds, sweet potatoes, wheat germ, avocados, and peanuts. A review of existing studies suggests that vitamin E's benefit in reducing heart attacks may not be seen unless it is used for more than two years, and probably at a dose greater than 100 IU (International Units). The recommended daily allowance of vitamin E is about 15 IU. Vitamin E may increase the risk of bleeding in some people.

The problem with many of these studies is that they are not comparing vitamin E use with a placebo. Instead, they are looking at the health of people who are taking the supplement, and comparing it to the health of people who are "vitamin-free." The criticism is that those taking the vitamin may live a healthier lifestyle in other ways — for example, they may jog more, eat less, or have more money in their bank accounts. To put it another way, vitamin use may be a marker of a healthier lifestyle as opposed to a contributor to the observed benefits of that lifestyle.

The routine use of vitamin E for the prevention of heart disease is widespread. I know many cardiologists who prescribe vitamin E for their patients and even take it themselves. Though there is mounting evidence that such advice is sound, there remains a wisp of uncertainty, and a fear that all patients will not gain so simply and easily. Perhaps the benefit is only seen in certain kinds of people. Maybe it is actually harmful in others. Studies of vitamin E have shown a slightly increased risk of bleeding in the brain, for example. It all depends how cautious one wishes to be and how much proof is required by the purist. I believe that the use of vitamin E has the **potential** to become as common and perhaps as useful a medication as aspirin for those with heart disease. There are many ongoing large trials to address this question further. My advice is to wait until the results are available (though I would never tell anyone not to take it).

Unproven Claims

Finally, **some** herbs and vitamins are clearly beneficial. Not all of them are. How do you as a consumer know which will help you and which will send you to an early grave? The only way is to test them rigorously. Patients expect this from drug companies; they should expect nothing less from vitamin and herb peddlars. It is not an issue of consumer choice but rather one of misleading the public with false health claims. I **am not** against herbs and vitamins because it erodes my "power base." I am not part of some giant physician-sponsored conspiracy to maintain control over the suffering populace. Elvis is dead, JFK was not assassinated by the CIA, and the world will (probably) not end in the year 2000. I **am** against duping the public with deceptions and distortions. There is nothing more important than one's health. Making a claim is easy. Proving it without bells, whistles, and lies is tough. So before you shell out big bucks for coenzyme Q10 or shark cartilage, think about whose health is really going to benefit — yours or the guy who sells the stuff.

POINTS TO REMEMBER

- **Vitamins and herbs do not have to be proven safe before they are marketed and sold.**

- Antioxidants (including many vitamins) are drugs which may reduce the risk of heart disease.

- Beta-carotene and vitamin A are antioxidants which are unhelpful in the prevention of heart disease and increase the risk of cancer in some people.

- Vitamin E is an antioxidant which appears to reduce the risk of heart attacks, but increases the risk of bleeding, including bleeding in the brain.

- Vitamin-rich foods are better (and cheaper) than vitamin-rich pills.

10

ALCOHOL & HEART DISEASE

It is rare for something considered pleasurable to have health benefits. The consumption of alcohol is demonized and coupled to social ills and physical ailments. Though we have seen alcohol prohibition attempted in this century, no attempts have been made to ban brussels sprouts, for example. This should not be misconstrued by brussels sprout farmers as an assault on their livelihood; however, most people don't plan their weekends around vegetables. ("Hey, Steve, what do you say we get a 12-pack of sweet potatoes and watch the ball game?") Alcoholism is an illness, so it is not surprising that most physicians shy away from prescribing it to prevent heart disease. Alcohol is a complex subject and we will restrict our discussion to its effects on the heart.

Many things in life are said to be beneficial in small amounts. Alcohol use is no exception. The effects of excess alcohol consumption can be quite serious and include liver failure and brain damage. Too much alcohol is toxic to the heart and can severely damage it. Physicians grade a patient's heart function on a four-point scale. This is typically done with a test known as an echocardiogram, which shows how strongly the heart beats. It employs the same technology (ultrasound) as that used to look at a pregnant woman's baby. Normal heart function is considered 1/4. When the heart muscle barely moves, it is called 4/4 dysfunction. Impaired function somewhere in the middle is 2/4 or 3/4. Prolonged alcoholism can result in 4/4 dysfunction. The chance of being alive one year after this problem is identified is under 50% if drinking continues. In some people, however, cessation of alcohol intake may normalize heart function, assuming alcohol was the cause of the problem in the first place.

Alcohol intake can affect the heart in other ways. If consumed in excess, it can cause holiday heart syndrome. In this disorder, patients arrive at hospitals, usually on weekend mornings, complaining of palpitations. They are found to have an irregular and rapid heartbeat called atrial fibrillation. Their history discloses excess alcohol use the night before. This interference with the heart's electrical system is usually transient unless alcohol use continues. Alcohol may also contribute to high blood pressure; reducing intake can be an effective way to lower it.

Now that we know a few of the evils of alcohol, what about the benefits? The answer is low to moderate alcohol ingestion **decreases** the risk of developing coronary artery

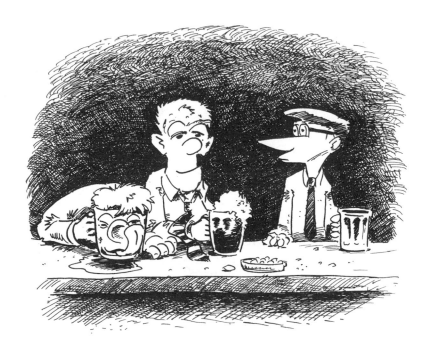

disease. Of course, if you do your drinking in smoke-filled bars with a hotdog in your mouth, you negate the potential benefits for your heart. This is not a license to get hammered out of your mind every day. I can just imagine a legion of drunkards stumbling around slurring that their doctor told them to get sloshed.

Figure 9 shows that the more you drink, the higher your mortality from such diverse conditions as cancer, stroke, and cirrhosis of the liver. Death rates increase for people who drink more than one or two alcoholic beverages per day. Drinkers who consume more than six beers at a sitting are more likely to topple over from a heart attack than those who stop at three. The data on the cardiac benefits of alcohol comes from observational studies totalling hundreds of thousands of people. One interesting study of nearly 100,000 nurses showed that those who drank an average of one and a half glasses of wine per day had nearly half the risk of coronary disease as those who drank no alcohol.

The benefits of alcohol are modest. Drinking one beer per night while ignoring other risk factors is comparable to eating a double hamburger, large fries, and milkshake, and chasing it down with a diet soft drink again. Although there has been a great deal of publicity about the benefits of red wine, the way in which these studies were scientifically conducted leaves room for doubt. Evidence suggests that white wine, beer, and spirits are equally beneficial to the heart. A recent study comparing red wine and vodka showed that only red wine was beneficial. Other studies have suggested that beer intake may **increase** the chances of developing coronary disease. At this time, however, the form in which alcohol is consumed (I mean wine, spirits, or beer, not liquid, solid, or gas) has not been rigorously examined to allow conclusive recommendations about the value of one over another.

The **"French paradox"** is a term used to describe the observation that though the French feast on fat-filled foods, their rates of coronary artery disease are low compared to

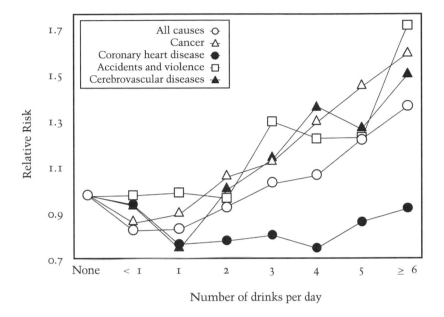

FIGURE 9

Alcohol consumption and relative risk of death over 12 years in the American Cancer Society study of 276,802 men ages 40 to 59 years.

most other industrialized nations. The study on which this is based dates from 1979. Although this may in part be due to the French's consumption of more alcohol than those in other countries, these observations may simply reflect under-reporting of cases of heart attacks. In other words, they may be cheating.

What exactly does a low to moderate intake of alcohol mean? Scientists describe intake in grams; but asking a bartender for 30 grams of beer or 20 grams of wine is unlikely to meet with understanding or service. The approximate level of alcohol consumption which protects against heart disease is 15 to 30 grams a day. This is equal to roughly one bottle of beer (a 12-ounce bottle, not a quart), one to two glasses of wine (a wineglass, not a pitcher), or one shot of the hard stuff (not the most you can swig from a bottle launched vertically over your mouth). Described another way, two to six drinks per week (not within an hour) produce the same desirable effects. Though this information represents some of the better studies on alcohol and heart disease, not all of the existing data fully supports these recommendations.

Women should know that even low doses of alcohol may slightly increase their risk of breast cancer. The recommendations for women are therefore more complex and should be individualized. Moderate drinking may also slightly increase the incidence of colon cancer, though this is uncertain.

The mechanisms by which alcohol exerts its benefits are probably a combination of many factors. For example, alcohol raises HDL, which is one of the most effective means of lowering cardiac risk. Alcohol also favourably alters LDL. But studies have suggested that only people with elevated LDL levels gain any cardiac benefit from alcohol consumption. Alcohol also has some anti-clotting ability which may prevent heart attacks.

Table 24
CARDIAC EFFECTS OF ALCOHOL
Benefits

1. Lower risk of coronary disease
2. Lower LDL levels
3. Higher HDL levels

Adverse effects

1. Heart muscle damage (prolonged, excessive use)
2. Holiday heart syndrome (rhythm disturbance called atrial fibrillation)
3. High blood pressure
4. Higher risk of colon cancer* (more than moderate use)
5. Higher risk of breast cancer

* debatable

So what is the bottom line? In those suffering from coronary artery disease, alcohol consumption may reduce future cardiac events. Selected patients who can responsibly handle the prescription should be encouraged to drink in the amounts discussed in this chapter. **Women should drink half this amount** because of the possibility of a slightly increased risk of breast cancer. It should be clear that these recommendations carry with them patient responsibility and accountability.

POINTS TO REMEMBER

- **Excessive alcohol use causes heart failure, high blood pressure, and heart rhythm problems.**
- **Small to moderate amounts of alcohol reduce the risk of heart disease.**
- **Alcohol raises HDL and lowers LDL.**
- **White wine, spirits, and beer are just as useful in lowering the risk of coronary artery disease as red wine.**
- **Women should drink less alcohol than men so as not to increase their risk of breast cancer.**

11

EXERCISE &
HEART DISEASE

Exercise is more than just the repetitive motion of body parts. The physical component is the easy part; the decision to get active is more difficult. The phrase "just do it" simplifies a complex subject. As with many aspects of health improvement, the issue is motivation.

Nearly 60% of North Americans are channel-surfing couch potatoes. Despite all of the fitness hype, only 1% of us regularly exercise. Lack of exercise is well established as an independent risk factor for the development of coronary artery disease. Though not as strong a risk as cigarette use or high blood pressure, a sedentary existence **doubles** the risk of developing heart disease.

The Benefits

In one study, 13,000 men and women were followed for eight years. The most physically fit people had the lowest death rates from heart disease. Another study of longshoremen (an example of an active job, though I'm not sure what they do) showed that they had less heart disease than the general population. Unfortunately, this protective effect was lost after about four years of resuming an inactive state. Thus, exercise is only protective if performed regularly. If you stop for a year, then your chance of heart disease is the same as all other couch potatoes. Another study of 5,000 Canadian government employees looked at their fitness levels and cardiac risk factors. Those workers who were the most physically fit also had the fewest cardiac risk factors. They had lower blood pressure, lower blood lipids, and weighed less than their unfit fellow workers. This suggests that being physically fit can have positive effects on your cardiac health.

Exercise will not extend a person's **maximum** lifespan, but it will reduce the chances of dying young. There is an average gain of four to seven years with regular exercise and good living habits. Other benefits of a consistent exercise routine include weight loss, improved blood sugar control in diabetics, reduction in the thinning of bones (osteoporosis), less colon and breast cancer, and "smoother" bowel habits. It is also of proven benefit in those with depression and anxiety. Exercise will not make you eat more than usual, though it has been shown to enhance the taste of food.

It amazes me what people call exercise. (Such as shown in the cartoon on the next page.) "Do you engage in a regular form of physical activity?" I ask my patients. "Sure," they respond. Only with closer scrutiny can I assess what people consider exercise. Sex (unless you are **very** active, **very** often) doesn't count. Nor does walking to the kitchen in between commercials, chasing the kids, or boating at the cottage, unless you're being dragged behind it. Exercise is more complex.

Static & Dynamic Exercise

Exercise can be either **static** or **dynamic**. Static exercise, also known as **isometrics**, includes weightlifting and involves muscles working against a fixed resistance for long periods of time. Dynamic exercise, or **isotonics**, involves repetitive lower resistance motion, important for developing endurance. Examples include running, swimming, cross-country skiing, etc. You may be able to swim for an hour, but even Mr. Universe (or Ms. Universe) can't lift 200 pounds

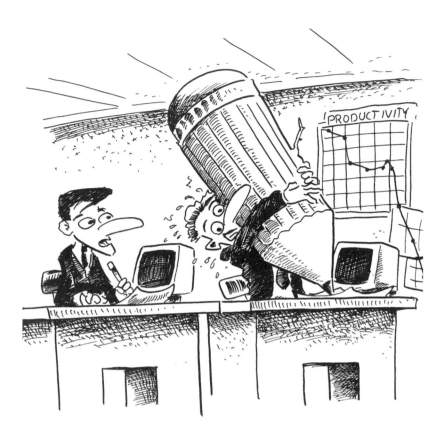

repeatedly over his head for too long. Static exercise is more likely to have unfavourable effects on blood pressure and is not recommended for patients with established heart disease. I'm not referring to light weights used for tone and strength, but rather heavier ones that make muscular people look like grapes constantly at risk of bursting through their skin. Aim for the raisin look.

Exercise has many beneficial effects on healthy and weak hearts include the development of larger and more numerous blood vessels (called **collaterals**). Exercise makes a diseased heart more electrically stable. Regular exertion also improves blood pressure, lowering both **systolic** (the higher number) and **diastolic** (the lower one) pressure. Exercise can overhaul blood lipid levels. It increases the level of good cholesterol (HDL) and decreases the level of bad cholesterol (LDL) and triglycerides. The modification of these risk factors is central to the beneficial effects of exercise.

Table 25

BENEFITS OF EXERCISE

1. Reduction in coronary artery disease
2. Reduction in blood pressure (systolic & diastolic)
3. Reduction in heart rate
4. Weight loss
5. Decrease in cholesterol
6. Decrease in LDL
7. Decrease in triglycerides
8. Increase in HDL
9. Larger and more numerous coronary artery branches
10. Improved sugar control
11. Less osteoporosis
12. Reduced incidence of breast cancer
13. Reduced incidence of colon cancer
14. Bowel regularity
15. Less depression
16. Less anxiety
17. Reduced likelihood of prematurely dying
18. Fewer colds

The Risks

Most of us have heard stories of people dropping dead during exercise. I have seen patients without vital signs brought to the emergency department in shorts and running shoes. Such sudden death is not just an anecdotal phenomenon, but rather a well-recognized risk of heavy exertion. **The hazard of sudden death is minuscule compared to the dangers of immobility.**

Obviously nothing is risk-free and both action and inaction can be deadly. Everyone's goal is to pursue the course with maximum benefit and minimum risk. The lowest risk category is **action**. While vigorously exercising, the risk of provoking a heart attack is up to five times higher compared to the risk in someone sitting there watching you. However, the **overall prognosis** of those who regularly exercise is three times better than that seated individual, even when you factor in the risk of a heart attack during exercise. In other words, that non-active person may be better protected during your hour of exercise, but it's the other 23 hours they need to worry about.

The risk of dying during exercise is greatest in previously inactive people who initiate a stressful program without prior preparation or physician assessment and guidance. The transient risk of a heart attack during intense exercise is 100 times higher in someone who isn't accustomed to vigorously exercising, and two to three times higher in someone who is accustomed to it. It is most likely to occur during the initial part of an exercise program in the elderly and in those with established cardiac disease.

There are more heart attacks after blizzards because of snow shovelling. More than 1,200 people in the United States die per year from heart attacks around the time of big snowstorms. If you have heart disease it's best to either pay your (younger) neighbour to clear your driveway or get your kid to do it.

The actual risk to patients with established heart disease (either a prior heart attack, previous bypass surgery, or coronary angioplasty) is extremely small. There is an average of one cardiac arrest (not always fatal) per 110,000 exercise hours, one heart attack per 300,000 exercise hours, and one death per 800,000 exercise hours. 300,000 hours is just over 34 years. The absolute risk of a 50-year-old non-diabetic nonsmoker provoking a heart attack during an hour of vigorous exercise is one in a million. The chance of dying during a jog is one per year per 7,620 **regular** joggers between ages 30 and 64. If you exclude those with known heart disease, the risk is one death per 15,240 joggers per year. This is per year, not per run.

It is very rare for healthy people without cardiac risk factors or symptoms to die while exercising. An interesting study did autopsies on 36 marathon runners who died suddenly during exercise. Twenty-seven (75%) had evidence of coronary artery narrowing, 75% had abnormal blood lipids, and 71% had prior warning symptoms. In a look at 75 recreational joggers over age 30 who died suddenly during exercise, 71 had narrowings in their coronary arteries. The message is that with a careful exercise program in which risk factors are closely assessed and monitored, the risk of suddenly dying during vigorous exertion is **much smaller** than the risk of not exercising.

Causes of Death During Exercise

The causes of sudden death during exercise are variable and depend on age. Older people who die during exercise are likely to have coronary artery disease. In a young person, however, sudden cardiac death is likely due to a congenital malformation in the heart. In other words, it is something he or she was born with. About half of cases of sudden death during exercise in young athletes are due to a well-described condition called **hypertrophic cardiomyopathy**. In this disease, the cells of the heart are abnormal and the heart muscle becomes extremely thick. This was the cause of death of Hank Gathers, a famous U.S. college player who died in 1990 within days of being drafted by the National Basketball Association.

There are a number of other famous athletes who have died during exertion. Pete Maravich, a player in the National Basketball Association, died during a pickup game of basketball, years after retiring. He was found to have had congenitally abnormal anatomy of his coronary arteries. Flo Hyman, an all-star volleyball player, died after a game in 1986. She ruptured her aorta, the main blood vessel coming from the heart. Jim Fixx, the fitness and jogging guru, died while running in 1984 at age 52. He had severe coronary artery disease. On the other hand, he also had high cholesterol, a family history of very premature heart disease, and was a heavy smoker until age 36. Reggie Lewis, another famous basketball player from the Boston Celtics, died suddenly while practising in Waltham, Massachusetts. He had previously collapsed on the court and been extensively investigated for heart disease. He may or may not have had a primary cardiac problem, and only the pathologist knows for sure.

Preparation

Anyone preparing to embark on an exercise program should first consult a physician and undergo a complete assessment of their cardiac risk factors. All men over 40 years of age and all women over 50 should undergo a treadmill test under physician guidance prior to starting a regular exercise program. The physical activity readiness questionnaire (PARQ) listed in table 26 can further assist decision-making. Beginning an exercise program in middle age still provides definite health benefits. It is never too late.

Once your doctor gives you the green light to exercise, a simple and common-sense approach is the way to go. A doctor told his patient that jogging 10 miles a day would improve his sex life and make him feel better. A week later, the doctor gets a phone call. "I feel great," his patient tells him. "Terrific," his doctor says. "What about your sex life?" "I don't know," the patient replies, "I'm 70 miles from home." It's unnecessary to jog 10 miles per day, unless you really want to. Lesser amounts of exercise will still provide benefit.

Table 26

PHYSICAL ACTIVITY
READINESS QUESTIONNAIRE (PARQ)

If you answer yes to any of the following questions, then any exercise, either informally or as part of a program, should be postponed until an assessment by a physician.

1. Have you ever been diagnosed with heart disease?
2. Do you often have chest pains?
3. Do you suffer from intense episodes of dizziness?
4. Have you ever been diagnosed with high blood pressure?
5. Do you have arthritis or other joint diseases which are worsened by exertion?
6. Is there any reason you should not pursue an exercise program, unrelated to the above questions?
7. Are you unaccustomed to regular exertion?

The Target Heart Rate

Regular exercise reduces the rate at which the heart beats during rest. This number is an indicator of fitness in healthy people. Those with lower heart rates at particular levels of exercise have a lower incidence of fatal heart disease. Highly trained athletes may have resting heart rates in the 30s. Heart rate decreases with age and certain drugs, so it shouldn't be used as the sole indicator of fitness.

The **target heart rate** can be used as a gauge of exercise intensity. You first have to know how to measure your heart rate. Simply feel for your radial artery pulse, which is at the wrist below your thumb with the palm facing upward. Count the number of pulsations over 15 seconds and multiply by four. The result is your heart rate per minute. To get your **maximum heart rate**, subtract your age from 220. The maximum heart rate is that achieved at the point of physical exhaustion. Unless you're a Marine (no offence to the other branches of the armed forces) or crazy, the maximum heart rate is not the goal. **The goal is the target heart**

rate, which is a percentage of the maximum heart rate. A target of 70–80% of your maximum rate for about 30 minutes or so is a good clip. For elderly patients, a target of 40–50% of the maximum heart rate is fine. The target is not the same for everyone at a particular age, and has an error of about 15 beats. If you calculate a target of 140 per minute and you feel fine exercising at 150, then exercise at 150. Simply follow logic. You shouldn't aim for your target at the start, but gradually work up to it. Concentrate more on getting a good workout for at least 30 minutes without pushing yourself to exhaustion in the first 10 minutes. Your heart rate is secondary to how you feel during your workout. You won't be able to maintain excessive heart rates for long periods of time. As you continue to exercise, the peak heart rate you achieve at the same level of exercise will actually decrease, reflecting improved fitness. If your jog resulted in a heart rate of 140 when you started exercising, after a few months you will find the same jog raises it to 120.

A Program

Exercise should include the following:

1. **Warm-up:** a 5–10 minute period used to limber up, improve flexibility, and reduce the chance of injury. The warm-up should slowly raise the heart rate and might include walking and stretching.
2. **Exercise:** should be done within the "target heart rate" for 30–60 minutes.
3. **Cool-down:** should occur over 5–10 minutes. During the cool-down period, the level of exertion should be slowly decreased.

Activity levels should follow three phases. Each phase comprises more exercise than the preceding one, and the resulting endurance is built up over months. The initial **conditioning** phase lasts about five weeks. During this time, one becomes accustomed to the type and intensity of exercise. This is followed by phase two, the **improvement** phase. It involves a gradual increase in the amount of exertion. This can last months as the amount of exercise is progressively increased toward the target level. **Maintenance levels** of exercise, the third phase, are achieved after about six months.

How Much Exercise?

How much exercise is required to really make a difference? The actual definitions, relating to oxygen use and energy expenditure, are best left to those who draw their salaries creating them. What the layperson needs is a practical guide to the amount of exercise necessary for cardiac benefit. To give a bit of scientific insight, the optimal amount of exercise results in a minimum of 4 kilocalories of energy expenditure per kilogram of body weight (4 kcal/kg). Inactivity only expends 1.5 of these kilocalories. Table 27 lists the energy expenditure associated with a whole array of activities. The more exercise performed, the greater the benefits. The more miles run per week, for example, the higher your levels of HDL, the good cholesterol. Triathlons, on the other hand, may be bad for the heart. They have been linked with heart damage due to the extreme and prolonged nature of those events.

Prescriptions for exercise include any of the following:

1. A brisk 2–3 km walk 3–5 times per week.
2. A 3-km in under 30 minutes 3–5 times per week.
3. A 3-km run in 30–40 minutes 6 days per week.

Frequency appears to be more important than duration. As you increase the frequency of vigorous exercise from one to five times per week, your chances of having a heart attack are progressively reduced. More than a half hour per session provides little additional benefit, however.

Table 27

ENERGY EXPENDITURE OF VARIOUS ACTIVITIES

Activity	Energy Expenditure (METS)
Sitting	1
Eating*	1.5

sitting & eating is not 2.5

Activity	Energy Expenditure (METS)
Washing dishes	2
Desk job	2
Driving	2
Walking slowly	2.5
Showering	3
Vacuuming	3
Bowling	3
Fishing	3
Shuffleboard	3
Bicycling at 10 km/hr	4
Gardening	4
Golfing (using a cart)	4
Walking briskly	5
Climbing stairs	5
Mowing the lawn	5
Bicycling at 15 km/hr	6
Golf (walking)	6
Dancing	6
Skating	6
Doubles tennis	6
Badminton	7
Jogging comfortably	8
Bicycling at 20 km/hr	8
Singles tennis	8
Shovelling snow	8
Swimming	8
Downhill skiing	9
Aerobics	9
Cross-country skiing	12
Jogging briskly	10–15
Sexual intercourse*	1–100

highly variable energy expenditure

A MET is a measure of energy expenditure. The standard reference is one MET. The longer an activity is done, the more METS used and calories burned.

Vigorous training is defined as enough to cause a sweat and a bit of breathlessness. Weight-bearing exercises such as walking, running, and cycling also reduce the chances of developing osteoporosis, though they increase the likelihood of orthopaedic injuries. Swimming, though not a weight-bearing form of exercise, is an excellent form of fitness. The chances of drowning are higher with swimming compared to golfing, unless you're an extremely obsessive all-weather player. Tennis is also an excellent form of exercise.

To the chagrin of many, regular exercise should be continued for at least five years to derive the full benefit. This should not discourage you from exercising. You will begin to see a myriad of gains after a very short time. It is always worth remembering that Finnish skiers have six to seven years of increased life expectancy above the general population, so the potential reward is large (especially if you live in Finland and like skiing). For ex-major-league football players, those who stopped exercising upon retirement had no evidence of benefit from their years of sweating it out. They simply became one of the masses when they stopped exercising. Their risk of developing heart disease was the same as the legions of people who never put on cleats and a jockstrap and never signed million-dollar contracts.

Colds

There is a relationship between colds and exercise. A cold is due to a virus, and results in symptoms including a sore throat, runny nose, headache, etc. The prevailing belief is that exercise protects athletes from such afflictions. The opposite actually occurs, at least with **extreme exertion**. Athletes who run more than 60 miles per week suffer from two times as many colds as those who run less than 20 miles per week. In a study of marathon runners, 13% had symptoms of a cold during the first seven days after the race, while only 2% reported symptoms before the race. Maybe all those people passing them cups of water along the route were also passing along germs. The risk of colds in saner people, who exercise moderately, is truly lower than those who don't exercise at all.

Sex

I wasn't sure where to put the sex section, but it seemed more closely related to exercise than fibre. Studies examining sexual activity after a heart attack (these were very nosy investigators!) have found that patients partake much less frequently after than before, so there is obviously concern about precipitating an event in the throes of passion. But studies show that the chance of provoking a heart attack during sex in a person who has had a prior heart attack is estimated at two in a million. These two people are presumably not in the same bed. This risk is no different in patients without heart disease. Considering the benefits, it seems silly to give it up, though you can do without the cigarette after. One proven method to reduce the danger is to exercise regularly. Think of it as a form of sexual training. **If a patient shows no evidence of problems during an exercise treadmill test, then he or she is very unlikely to have problems during sex.**

In half the cases of death during sex, the cause is not heart related. Interestingly, when the heart is implicated, the event often occurs during intercourse with someone other than the spouse. In a study of 5,559 fatal heart attacks, 18 were during intercourse, and 14 of these were during sex with someone other than the wife or husband. This is not a moral dissertation on extramarital affairs; however, if you're caught, death at the hands of your spouse is not the only way you could go.

The demands sex places on the heart depend upon the energy expended, and some people expend more energy than others. For the typical married adult, sex modestly increases heart rate and blood pressure. If you have sex with someone other than your spouse, the increases may be far from modest. The energy costs of sex are comparable to ascending two flights of stairs (I'd like to see the research techniques of that study), so if you can do one you should be able to do the other. Engaging in sex while climbing stairs is not recommended, though on stairs is acceptable (if they are carpeted). Though hot-tub use has been investigated and found to be safe in patients with stable angina, "activities" in hot tubs should be avoided in patients with heart disease.

You can decrease your cardiac risk during sexual intercourse by choosing a familiar environment (not an airplane washroom no matter how familiar it is), being well rested, and abstaining from alcohol or heavy meals a few hours before. Your heart rate and blood pressure are not that different during intercourse than during other daily activities. Even patients with angina should be able to partake with pleasure and without worry.

POINTS TO REMEMBER

- **Lack of exercise is a risk factor for heart disease. Exercising will reduce that risk and lower blood pressure, weight, and lipids.**

- **Your chance of having a problem with exercise is a lot less than your chance of having a problem without it.**

- **Before starting an exercise routine, have your physician do a stress test to make sure it's safe.**

- **There are many different exercise routines. Choose one that keeps you at your target heart rate long enough to build up a sweat and cause mild breathlessness.**

- **Always allow logic to prevail when it comes to type and duration of exercise. Build up to a maintenance level gradually over months.**

- **If you can climb two flights of stairs, you should be able to engage in sexual intercourse without fear of a sudden heart attack.**

I2

HIGH BLOOD PRESSURE

Blood pressure, or BP, means exactly what it sounds like. It is the pressure generated by the heart to propel blood through the body. Also known as **hypertension**, high blood pressure is a leading cause of cardiovascular disease in North America. It is a major risk factor for heart attacks and strokes. About 15% of people have hypertension and 40% of those over 60 suffer from it.

Think of the pressure which drives water through a fire hose. The hose represents the **blood vessels**, the water represents blood, and the pump generating the pressure is the **heart**. If a fire was limited to the fourth floor of a building, then firemen on the street would need a certain water pressure to douse the flames. Anything less and the water would not reach the target. Excessive pressure would allow the water to reach higher floors and would be an unnecessary expenditure. If the fire hose was trained on the building for a long time, damage could result. Perhaps a wall would collapse. Blood pressure is the same in that a certain amount is required to move blood through the body. Hypertension is too much pressure. If the organs are exposed to too much pressure over time, then like a wall exposed to a constant high-pressure water stream, damage can result. **The higher the blood pressure, the more work the heart is performing. The harder the heart muscle works, the more likely it is that coronary artery disease and heart failure will develop.**

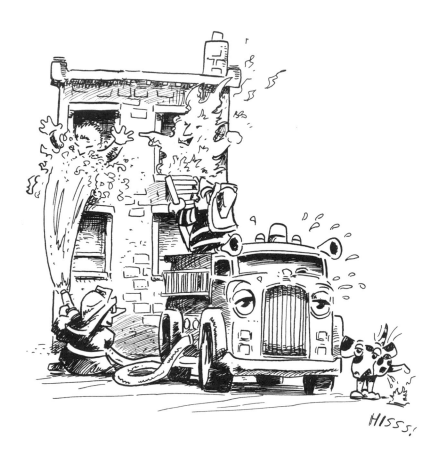

HISSS!

Systolic & Diastolic

Blood pressure is reported as two numbers, for example 120 over 80 (120/80). The "top" number (120 in this case) is called the **systolic pressure**. The "bottom" number is the **diastolic pressure**. Elevation of *either or both* is hypertension. The systolic pressure is the pressure measured in the blood vessels with **each** heartbeat. Diastolic pressure is the pressure in the blood vessels when the heart relaxes **between** beats. Clench your fist (about the size of your heart) and this generates systolic pressure. When your fist relaxes, it is the diastolic pressure. Each is a measurement of the actual pressure within the blood vessels.

Symptoms & Signs

Hypertension is often referred to as a silent killer. There is usually a lag period of decades from the onset of high blood pressure until the symptoms appear. During this time people may be completely unaware that they have hypertension. It may not produce symptoms until irreversible damage occurs. Hypertension is most often diagnosed in an unsuspecting patient during a routine visit to the doctor's office. Symptoms which **may** reflect high blood pressure include headaches, nose bleeds, dizziness, frequent urination at night, and excessive tiredness. However, most of these complaints are due to some other cause. These symptoms should prompt a visit to a physician, though there will usually be a simple explanation.

High blood pressure is a major risk factor for coronary artery disease, strokes, heart failure, and blindness, and is the leading cause of kidney failure. Prolonged (i.e., over many years) hypertension damages blood vessels, creating a fertile milieu for the formation of coronary artery disease. It does the same to blood vessels supplying the brain, resulting in an increase in debilitating strokes (what other kind are there?). This is why hypertension recognition and control is so important. The earlier it is recognized, the more likely it is that its deadly effects can be prevented.

Hypertension is **primary** 90–95% of the time. This means there is no identifiable cause. In the other 5–10%, hypertension is **secondary** to another disease. There are many diseases which can cause high blood pressure. A partial list is supplied in table 28.

What Is High Blood Pressure?

Elevations in diastolic and/or systolic pressure are defined as hypertension. Both are associated with complications. A single blood pressure elevation, unless extremely elevated, is insufficient to establish the diagnosis of high blood pressure. There must be multiple elevations on readings taken months apart. Some physicians recommend three to five measurements over six months, while others will make the diagnosis with two measurements over a two-week period. A middle ground likely achieves the same goal.

Table 28

CAUSES OF HIGH BLOOD PRESSURE*

1. Kidney disease
2. Adrenal gland disease
3. Thyroid disease
4. Steroids (prednisone, birth control pills, and anabolic steroids)
5. Pregnancy may be the first time high blood pressure is detected
6. Narrowing of the aorta (called "coarctation")
7. Sleep apnea
8. Alcohol/drug use (cocaine)
9. Leakiness of the aortic valve
10. Some prescription drugs

*This is not an exhaustive list. There are a multitude of other causes of high blood pressure, though many of them are rare.

What values constitute hypertension?

1. A diastolic pressure under 90 and a systolic pressure under 140 are **normal**.

2. A diastolic pressure of 90–104 is **mild hypertension**.

3. A diastolic pressure more than 104 is **moderate hypertension**.

4. A diastolic pressure more than 114 is **severe hypertension**.

5. A systolic pressure of 140–160 is classified as **borderline hypertension**.

6. A systolic pressure over 160 is definitive and a systolic over 160 with diastolic of less than 90 is called **isolated systolic hypertension**.

White Coat Hypertension

A separate entity worth mentioning is **white-coat hypertension**. If blood pressure is elevated in the doctor's office but normal at other times, for example on a home monitor or at the gym, then white-coat hypertension may be present. Doctors make many people nervous. (They make *me* nervous.) An elevation in blood pressure is an understandable result of anxiety. The best response is not complete avoidance of your physician. If suspected, **ambulatory blood pressure monitoring** may be diagnostic. This is a small machine to take home which periodically measures blood pressure over 24 hours. If ambulatory BP measurements are normal, then the hypertension measured in the office is white-coat. Home blood pressure monitors will set you back about $100. They are useful in monitoring your blood pressure in the comfort of your home, unless your loved ones raise your blood pressure more than your doctor. Drug therapy is rarely indicated for white-coat hypertension.

Who is most likely to develop hypertension? The incidence of hypertension increases with age. As with nearly all cardiac disease, men are more likely to develop hypertension than women. Blacks have a higher incidence than other races, and tend to develop complications more often. People in the former Soviet Union have been found to have very high levels of blood pressure, possibly related to alcohol use and stress.

Who Is at Risk?

What are some of the risks which predispose to hypertension and how can they be modified? Though there are a number of factors which increase the chances of developing high blood pressure, it may occur in otherwise healthy individuals for no obvious reason. Doctors tend to chalk this up to genetics, which often becomes a grab bag for things we don't yet understand.

Age is a risk; however it is non-modifiable. A history of blood pressure elevation in a parent or sibling doubles your chances of developing it. Obesity is associated with high blood pressure. The heavier a person is, the more likely they will develop it. A sedentary existence is also a risk factor. The more time spent at a desk, on a couch in front of the television, or at a desk in front of a couch, the more likely it is that blood pressure will rise. Salt ingestion is correlated with high blood pressure, as is alcohol use. The more you drink, the more likely it is that hypertension will develop, though the less likely it is that you will care. Caffeine intake does not contribute to hypertension. The workplace can affect blood pressure. Emergency room physicians are more likely to have higher readings when on the job, probably due to the high stress environment. Hypertension is also associated with frequent exposure to loud noise.

SWEAR

The decision to treat hypertension is based on many variables. As with other diseases, there are effective therapeutic options which **do not utilize drugs**. If these work, great. Medications are usually more effective in controlling blood pressure, though, and if it remains elevated despite alternative approaches, drugs should be started. By alternative, I mean approaches with **proven** potential benefit, not **claimed** benefit. Certain drugs will definitely save lives by reducing the blood pressure, and with it events like heart attacks and strokes. Some people make the mistake of taking their **antihypertensives** (drugs which lower blood pressure) only when they feel unwell. High blood pressure is almost always silent. If you feel well, it does not mean your blood pressure is normal. These drugs are ineffective when used episodically.

The acronym I employ for non-drug therapy of hypertension is SWEAR:

S = salt. Some people with hypertension respond dramatically to salt restriction. Older patients with high blood pressure are more likely to respond than younger people with normal blood pressure. Other studies claim that a diet low in salt may help **prevent** hypertension in most people, regardless of age or blood pressure levels. Though not a cure, current evidence supports restricting salt intake whether you have normal or elevated readings.

Table 29

SALT SOURCES

1. Table salt
2. Processing & cooking
3. Naturally present in some foods

Vegetables High in Salt

1. Beets
2. Carrots
3. Spinach
4. Celery
5. Rutabagas
6. White Turnips
7. Kale

Processed Goods High in Salt

1. Almost all processed meats, fish, and cheese
2. Salted snacks (chips, crackers, popcorn, nuts, pretzels)
3. Sauces, dressings, condiments (except spices, herbs, etc.)
4. Frozen, pickled, and packaged foods
5. Canned foods (soups and vegetables)
6. Some laxatives, antacids, and mouthwashes

Salt (also known as sodium and abbreviated as Na^+) should be used sparingly in cooking and should not be added from the table shaker (or bowl or dish or saucer). Foods high in salt should be avoided (table 29). Most of our dietary salt is on the plate before it arrives at the table, so shunning the salt shaker does not necessarily translate into a low salt diet. Foods high in salt include processed meats, canned goods, fast foods, and a myriad of other products. Reading packages should become routine and is the best way to avoid sodium-laden meals. The closer it is to the top of the ingredient list, the more salt a product contains. There are a number of salt substitutes which some people find palatable, though others are less generous in their assessments.

W = weight. Weight reduction through diet and exercise definitely reduces blood pressure. A diet high in fruits, vegetables, low fat dairy products, and fibre, and low in saturated fats, is associated with rapid (i.e., weeks) and significant blood pressure reduction. Vegetarians have lower blood pressure than meat eaters.

E = exercise. Patients who exercise briskly three to four times per week for 20–30 minutes not only lose weight but also reduce blood pressure.

A = alcohol. Though some alcohol protects against heart disease, too much will raise blood pressure. One drink per day should not be exceeded very often. This does not mean that you can stay on the wagon for six days and get drunk on day seven.

R = relaxation. When I talk to patients in my office about reducing their blood pressure, I mention the potential value of stress reduction. Though the benefits have not been as clearly demonstrated as with exercise, learning to relax won't hurt. It is difficult to give advice about relaxation. Most of us would prefer to live stress-free, but our individual realities quickly diverge from this ideal. Most doctors are not adequately trained in relaxation techniques, such as biofeedback, yoga, transcendental meditation, or tai chi. If patients wish to reduce their stress, or if I believe this would be useful, I will refer them to the appropriate professional.

Hypertension is a complex risk factor. Despite extensive research, there remains much to be discovered. That high blood pressure is a major killer is an unassailable fact. That treating high blood pressure reduces heart attacks, strokes, and death is equally certain. A combination of lifestyle changes and medication is essential for anyone with this disease. Don't be fooled by the absence of easily recognized and tangible proof of high blood pressure. Like a lion silently stalking a gazelle, it will kill you before you know it is lurking.

POINTS TO REMEMBER

- **High blood pressure is a major risk factor for coronary artery disease, kidney failure, stroke, and blindness, and, like a parasite, has usually been with you a while before you realize it.**

- **High blood pressure may be systolic, diastolic, or both, and all forms are dangerous.**

- **For some people, blood pressure is only high at the doctor's office, or particularly uncontrolled when measured by a physician. If ambulatory blood pressure measurements confirm elevated numbers, it is worth investing in a good home monitor.**

- **Non-drug ways to lower blood pressure should be actively pursued (see "SWEAR").**

- **If SWEAR doesn't reduce your blood pressure, then you should be started on medications (anti-hypertensives).**

13

MENOPAUSE & HEART DISEASE

Menopause (more than simply a pause) is an equalizer of men and women in the realm of cardiac disease. Prior to menopause, coronary artery disease is uncaringly sexist, as men are much more likely to suffer from it in their thirties and forties than are women. This is the cost of the male hormone testosterone coursing through our veins. In the absence of multiple cardiac risk factors like high blood pressure, diabetes, abnormal lipids, and cigarettes, it is unusual for women to suffer from angina or heart attacks before menopause. This represents a benefit of the hormone estrogen. The only other animal which undergoes menopause is the pilot whale.

There is enough literature on estrogen and menopause to stock an entire bookstore, and I'm sure there's such a store out there somewhere. The goal of this chapter is to discuss the cardiac effects of menopause, the beneficial and adverse effects of estrogen therapy, and the controversy surrounding its use. There are multiple reasons for initiating hormonal therapy in post-menopausal women. The prevention of coronary disease is the most compelling. When estrogen production declines, heralding the onset of menopause, the rate of coronary artery disease in women begins to catch up to that of men. These rates equalize for men and women by age 75. Women older than 55 have 10 times the rate of CAD compared to women aged 35–54.

Estrogen is a hormone produced in large amounts in the ovaries and in smaller amounts in the adrenal glands. The adrenal glands are peanut-sized organs which sit atop the kidneys like berets. The ovaries are the female version of the testicles (or alternatively the testicles are the male version of the ovaries). Men produce small amounts of estrogen from the adrenal glands as well, though most wouldn't admit it. Estrogen is also produced by fat cells in the body. This is why overweight women are less likely to have symptoms of menopause than slimmer women.

What Is Menopause?

As women approach the crest of middle age, estrogen production gradually declines, then ceases until the ovaries no longer release eggs. When estrogen production begins this decline, a woman is said to have entered menopause. Estrogen production stops (and menopause starts) in one of two ways. Most commonly it occurs **naturally** as a woman ages. Alternatively, a woman may have her ovaries **surgically** removed (called an oophorectomy), perhaps as part of a hysterectomy (removal of the uterus). Many women who undergo this procedure are unaware that their ovaries have also been removed. Whether natural or surgical, the health implications of ovarian failure are the same.

Menopause can be defined in a number of ways. It may start after a woman's final menstrual period, or alternatively, at the cessation of menstruation for more than a year. Menopause occurs at an average age of 51, but may occur earlier or later. It is more likely to be a few years premature in smokers.

Symptoms & Signs of Menopause

Menopause is a gradual process, occurring over an average of five years. Some women go through it in 10 years but for others, it lasts only months. Estrogen deficiency accounts for nearly all of the symptoms of menopause. Initial complaints begin weeks to months after estrogen production starts to wane. These include hot flashes, night sweats, insomnia, dry skin, depression, irritability, and mild memory loss.

Additional symptoms occur later and are related to the loss of estrogen's effects on certain tissues. There may be vaginal dryness, resulting in painful intercourse. Urinary incontinence and frequent urination are also common complaints. Unfortunately, wrinkles are more likely to occur with menopause. This is partly from the loss of estrogen's effects on the skin. The most serious consequences of menopause are gradual, and occur over decades. For example, the density of bone decreases (osteoporosis), which increases the incidence of fractures. More importantly, the cardiovascular system is no longer as well protected from atherosclerosis, leading to an increased likelihood of angina and heart attacks.

Table 30

MENOPAUSE — SIGNS & SYMPTOMS

Early (weeks to months)

Hot flashes	Depression
Dry skin	Irritability
Night sweats	Mild memory loss
Insomnia	

Later (months to years)

Coronary artery disease	Bone fractures
Urinary incontinence	Weight gain
Frequent urination	Elevated cholesterol
Vaginal dryness	Elevated LDL
Wrinkles	Elevated triglycerides
Osteoporosis	Reduced HDL

Menopause has a number of important effects on lipids. Unfortunately, all of them are negative. The cessation of estrogen production throws a woman's lipid profile into turmoil. When estrogen production grinds to a halt, the liver becomes less efficient at chewing up cholesterol. As more cholesterol is free to roam the blood vessels, **total cholesterol and LDL increase and HDL decreases**. Triglycerides also increase, though the effect is negligible. Cholesterol actually slowly creeps up years **before** menopause begins. As we are on the subject of fat, women tend to gain weight after menopause, initially averaging about a pound and a half per year. This trend can be combatted with the familiar duo of diet and exercise.

Herbs, Vitamins, & Menopause

So what can be done to combat the symptoms of menopause, and what are the benefits and risks of beginning estrogen and progesterone replacement? Menopause represents a lush market for herbal remedies. One hot item is **Oil of Evening Primrose capsules**. Lyrical name, lovely package, aromatic fragrance, and absolutely useless. In well-designed studies, these capsules have been compared with placebo. This herbal remedy has been found to be **ineffective** in treating the symptoms associated with menopause, so don't rely on anecdotal advocacy; save your money. If 25% of women feel better taking nothing but sugar pills (this is called the **placebo effect**), then the same may be true of an ineffective drug such as Oil of Evening Primrose. Therefore, just because someone says, "It works for me," doesn't mean that it is an effective therapy. Acupuncture has been touted as a treatment for the hypertension that accompanies menopause. Other than leaving you with needles in your body, it is ineffective for this purpose according to numerous studies. I would love it if these things worked, but the contents of the bottle should be more important than the package it comes in, including the marketing package.

The same is true of **vitamin E**, another popular "alternative" offering for hot flashes. It has been studied in a randomized, blinded, controlled study. No better than sugar pills. As for **ginkgo biloba** (sounds like a reptile or a contender in boxing's lightweight division), **vitamin B6** and **antioxidants**, I have three words: unproven, unproven, and unproven (that's four words). They may work, but it has never been studied. Gingko is associated (rarely) with serious spontaneous bleeding and tremendous wealth (commonly) for those marketing it as a cure-all. Its uses are limited, though it may mildly reduce the progression of dementia.

Another booming supplement is **phytoestrogens**, which are plant forms of estrogen. As with most supplements, phytoestrogens have been subject to negligible safety testing. They have been effectively marketed as natural, drawing scores of people onto the herbal bandwagon. Once again, just because it is derived from plants does not make it benign. That is a dangerous assumption. Mushrooms are "natural" but some varieties will kill you. There is no research available on the safety or usefulness of phytoestrogens, merely anecdotes from people who stand to make loads of money off of them. Estrogen use without progesterone promotes uterine cancer. How do we know that phytoestrogens don't increase the risk of uterine cancer? We don't. Though I hope we may one day advocate many natural drugs, like aspirin for example, I think it is safer to find out which ones will kill you and which ones will help you live longer **before** peddling them.

The Benefits of Hormone Therapy

So what can hormone replacement therapy with estrogen and **progesterone** (another hormone produced by the ovaries) do for you? Estrogen replacement has been shown to prevent osteoporosis, which accompanies menopause. It will not reverse bone loss which has already occurred, so the earlier estrogen is used, the better. It may also reduce the risk of developing Alzheimer's dementia, lower the

Estrogen and progesterone use in menopausal women will improve a woman's lipid profile. LDL is significantly reduced, and HDL is increased. This is only true if the hormones are taken in pill form. When estrogen is administered by other routes, including skin patches, its beneficial effects on the lipid profile are less.

Estrogen therapy for post-menopausal women without a history of coronary heart disease results in improvement in all forms of cardiovascular disease, including a reduction in angina, heart attacks, and strokes. This is in bold letters for obvious reasons. Estrogen decreases death and illness from coronary artery disease by about 50% if used for more than five years. Recent publication of the Hormone Estrogen Replacement Trial (HERS) has modified our approach to HRT in women with a history of CAD. This study enrolled nearly 3,000 women with heart disease and randomized them to HRT or placebo. In the first year of the study, slightly more women either had heart attacks or died in the HRT group compared to the placebo group! In the ensuing three years of the study, the opposite was true. Therefore, though HRT seems to benefit otherwise healthy women without heart disease, it may increase the risk of problems in older women with heart disease during the first year of use. The big question is why. We know that hormone replacement therapy may increase the likelihood of clots forming in blood vessels. Remembering that a blood clot is the ultimate cause of a heart attack, HRT in women with heart disease may promote blood clots in already diseased arteries. After a year, however, the beneficial effects of HRT, for example a reduction in cholesterol, outweigh the risks.

Because women taking HRT for more than a year had fewer heart attacks, the increased risk during the first year may be "worth it" in the long run. Unfortunately we simply do not know the right answer in this particular group of women. Therefore initiating HRT in older women with established heart disease cannot be recommended at this time. It may still be beneficial in the long term, but such women need to understand the potential risk during initial use, before they decide to take HRT.

The cardiac rewards of hormone therapy are lost within five years of stopping estrogen. Estrogen has no demonstrable effect when used by women over 75 years old and it **increases** the rates of coronary artery disease in men.

Progesterone plays various roles in the body. When estrogen is used without progesterone, the rate of uterine cancer increases. This is especially true when high dosages of estrogen are used (more than 0.625 mg of conjugated estrogen). However when progesterone is taken in addition to estrogen, the increased risk of uterine cancer is eliminated. If a dosage of 5–10 mg is used for at least 12 days per month, the risk of uterine cancer will actually **decrease**. Though the use of progesterone has been found to counteract a few of estrogen's beneficial effects on the lipid profile, these changes are not significant in low doses. If a woman has had her uterus removed, progesterone is unnecessary.

There are many potential side effects from estrogen use, some harmless and others life-threatening. The most common is mastalgia, a confusing way of saying breast pain. This usually resolves within three months of initiating therapy. Another effect is an increased sex drive. There is no way to comment on this delicately, so I will let it lie. Menstruation, an unwelcome reminder of youth for many women, may return when hormone therapy is started. It usually abates within a year for most women. Estrogen use also increases the incidence of gallstones twofold.

Estrogen Use & Breast Cancer

These are mostly asides. The major concern for women is the purported association between estrogen supplements and breast cancer. The suggestion that estrogen use may increase the risk of breast cancer is of enormous concern to all post-menopausal women considering hormone replacement therapy. When the data from multiple studies is mixed in the same cauldron, there is an increased risk of developing breast cancer when estrogen is used for more than 10 to 15 years. This risk has not been shown to increase from short-term use of less than five years, and rather inexplicably, there is reduced risk of dying from breast cancer in short-term users of estrogen. But these studies are not without flaws. Some of them used **twice** the usual dose of estrogen and in others, the types of estrogen studied are no longer used. Conjugated estrogen, the most commonly used preparation, has not been associated with an increased incidence of breast cancer. Most studies which have suggested an increased risk of breast cancer are methodologically unsound. A number of more recent trials, involving tens of thousands of women, show very little increased risk of breast cancer at all. One involved more than 100,000 women and concluded that there was no increased risk of dying in women who develop breast cancer while on hormone replacement.

The increased risk of cardiovascular disease in post-menopausal women not on hormone replacement must be weighed against the negligible chance of developing breast cancer. Let's put this risk in a statistical perspective. **Between the ages of 50 and 94, 31% of all deaths in women are attributed to coronary artery disease**, and nearly a third of these deaths occur before the age of 65. A further 3% of women in this age range die from hip fractures. About 3% of women between 50 and 94 die from breast cancer. Even if hormone replacement therapy caused a very small increase in breast cancer, the reduction in heart disease, decrease in bone loss, and improved muscle strength suggests it should be used when not contraindicated.

Let's look at the statistics in another way. Women older than 50 on hormone therapy for over five years increase their risk of breast cancer from 45 cases per 1,000 women to 47 cases (that's two extra cases). If used for more than 10 years, the risk rises to 51 cases per 1,000 (six more), and if used for over 15 years, 57 cases (12 more). After a woman has been off hormone therapy for five years, the risk of breast cancer is no different than for someone who never took it. Breast cancer in women on hormone therapy is also more likely to be smaller and easier to treat. On the other side of the scale, the use of hormone replacement protects 55 of every 1,000 women (that's 55 cases) from cardiac disease and five from serious bone fractures.

There are studies underway which may modify our present approach to hormone replacement therapy. There are no simple equations to identify an individual's risks and benefits from hormone use. It remains a personal and informed decision based on a woman's concerns and fears of each disease, as well as one's personal and family history of breast cancer. The most recent study of this subject, however, shows that women on estrogen who have a family history of breast cancer are not at any increased risk of developing it.

I believe that in most situations, hormone replacement therapy should be used. There are instances in which it may not be the right choice, though only about 1% of healthy post-menopausal women should not be on hormone replacement. If a woman has an increased risk of breast cancer by virtue of a personal or family history and a low risk of heart disease, it may not be appropriate to use, though even this has not been adequately sorted out.

The chance a woman will develop breast cancer in her life is 12%, or roughly one in eight. Breast cancer is so frighteningly common that many women on hormone replacement therapy will develop it regardless of their decision about estrogen use. Anecdotal reports of breast cancer developing while on hormones should never be given much weight. As with all aspects of health care, decisions must reflect informed opinion. There is no corner on the information market. It often takes surprisingly little research, such as reading a chapter in a book for example, to learn enough details to make intelligent choices. I approach my patients as if they are my relatives and think, What would I advise my relative to do? When it comes to estrogen, I believe it should be used in women without a history of coronary heart disease.

POINTS TO REMEMBER

- When a woman enters menopause, she no longer produces estrogen and progesterone. Among many other effects, her risk of heart disease skyrockets.

- Though many herbal remedies are marketed as menopause cure-alls, none has been proven to be better than placebo.

- Estrogen supplementation must always be used with progesterone in women who have not had hysterectomies (removal of uterus), due to the increased risk of uterine cancer with estrogen alone.

- Hormone therapy greatly reduces coronary artery disease, bone loss, and muscle weakness. It also decreases other effects of aging and increases sex drive.

- For almost all women, the increased risk of breast cancer is small and pales in comparison to the cardiac benefits for almost all women without coronary heart disease.

14

TOBACCO & HEART DISEASE

Everyone (especially tobacco company executives) knows that smoking increases the risk of dying. Not everyone will admit it (you know who you are), but everyone knows it. Tobacco is a product which when used as suggested will cause cancer, heart attacks, and a multitude of other ailments. According to the U.S. Surgeon General, smoking is "the chief single avoidable cause of death in our society." Insurance firms, some of which are actually owned by tobacco companies, charge smokers higher rates for life insurance. The purpose of this section is to get you to quit before you hack out an entire lung onto the dinner table.

Risks

In Canada, there are over 100 deaths per day from smoking-related disease. Worldwide, there is a death every 13 seconds due to a smoking-related illness (not exactly every 13 seconds, but on average). About 25% of North Americans over 15 years of age smoke and one in five will die as a result. Level of education is one predictor of cigarette use. College graduates are less likely to smoke (16%) compared to high school dropouts (36%). Knowledge of the perils of smoking does not confer immunity from the habit. Up to 10% of Canadian physicians smoke. This contrasts with 15% of lawyers and 27% of nurses. In Japan and France, about 40% of physicians smoke.

It's always interesting to hear a tale about the 90-year-old great-grandmother who smokes two packs of cigarettes per day and runs the Boston Marathon in less than four hours. Many smokers earnestly quote such anecdotal tales of longevity to justify the safety of the habit. "My grandfather died at the age of 106 and smoked four packs of cigarettes per day, so it can't be bad for you." If 100 pedestrians crossed a busy highway during rush hour, the testimony of the 10 survivors wouldn't be used as an indication of the safety of the trek. No physician ever claimed that everyone who smokes will die. Smokers simply have a greater statistical chance of developing a gruesome disease (table 31).

Table 31

SMOKING

Adverse effects	Benefits
1. Coronary artery disease	
2. Heart attacks	
3. Cancer (name an organ, any organ)	
4. Strokes	
5. Peripheral vascular disease	
6. Emphysema	
7. Asthma	
8. Miscarriages	
9. Infertility	
10. Low birth weight	
11. Childhood asthma	
12. Childhood pneumonia	
13. Ear infections	
14. Sudden infant death	
15. Early childhood death	
16. Bad teeth	
17. Bad breath	
18. Wrinkles	
19. Early menopause	

Smoking increases your risk of heart attacks, strokes, lung cancer, debilitating lung disease, and a potpourri of other

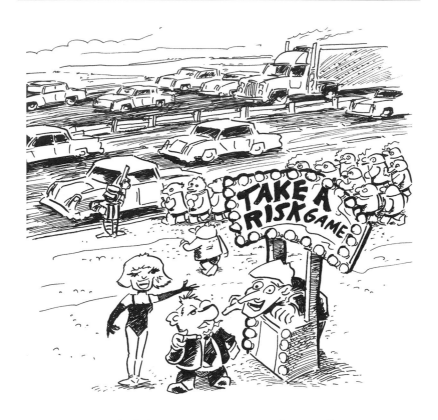

*"And if you win, your prize is that you'll
get to tell your grandchildren about it."*

nasty afflictions. It would be easy to drag out that statement and focus on the horrors of each disease, but what for? The evidence is so overwhelming that only someone with a financial interest in tobacco or a serious nicotine addiction would claim smoking is safe. This is an oversimplification. Smoking is not a logical form of leisure. No amount of statistical babble will convert the unconverted. If an informed individual chooses to smoke, neither coercion, pleadings, nor threats will change his or her mind. The personal choice to smoke should be respected — as long as it is undertaken outdoors, of course.

Though our focus is the effects of smoking on the cardio-vascular system, there are important non-cardiac effects.

Lung cancer is the leading cause of cancer death among men and women in North America (30% of all cancer deaths). Over 90% of lung cancer is directly attributable to smoking. This allows legions of smokers to loudly proclaim that people who don't smoke still get lung cancer. Some people survive plane crashes, too, but I wouldn't get on one if there was a 20% chance of dying on each flight.

Though there is never a good time to start, the long-term effects of smoking are dependent on the age at which you take your first drag. Smokers who begin before the age of 15 have four times the incidence of lung cancer compared to those who start after age 25. More than 80% of adult smokers took up the addiction before their twenty-first birthday. The peak age is 16.

Medicine often talks about five-year survival rates as a gauge of the impact and prognosis of any disease. The five-year survival rate of primary lung cancer is a mere 15%. At the end of five years, 85 out of every 100 people diagnosed with lung cancer are dead. What do we mean by primary? All cancer is classified as either primary or secondary. A **secondary** (metastatic) tumor is one that did not arise where it was discovered. For example, a piece of a liver tumor under the microscope may be a lung cancer which has spread to the liver. The liver mass is classified as a secondary or metastatic tumor. A primary tumor is one which started in the organ in which it was identified.

Through a condition called **emphysema**, smoking destroys lung tissue with debilitating effects. Imagine feeling as if you've run a race each time you go to the washroom or walk to the car. The effects of smoking are dose-related. The more you smoke, the more likely it is you'll get a terrible disease. Heavy smokers (more than 25 cigarettes per day) increase their risk of emphysema by 30 times. Light smokers can't feel safe, either. Women who smoke one to four cigarettes per day have a two and a half times higher rate of fatal heart disease. Those who smoke more than 25 cigarettes per day have five and a half times the risk. Smoking has been linked to ovarian, cervical, uterine, and bladder cancer. There is also a connection between cigarettes and breast cancer.

Denial is medically omnipotent. I've seen many patients and families who remain convinced to the final day that the lung cancer which has entered their lives had nothing to do with the two-pack-a-day smoking habit. The issue of taking personal responsibility for health never enters their minds. Attempting education once a fatal illness has taken hold is sadistic.

Cigars

Cigars and pipes are thought of as less likely to cause cancer than cigarettes. This depends on the amount smoked. The nicotine in cigars is no less addictive than that found in cigarettes, though few people smoke 20 cigars a day. In Holland and Denmark, the rate of lung cancer from pipes and cigars is similar to that from cigarettes. The difference is that the Dutch and Danes inhale the smoke from pipes and cigars more deeply. Cigar smokers have a 34% higher rate of cancer than abstainers. Second-hand cigar smoke is even more toxic than cigarette emissions. Celebrities such as Wayne Gretzky and Arnold Schwarzenegger encourage and promote cigar use with their appearances in magazines supporting the industry. Would they encourage their own children to puff on a fat cancer stick? I doubt it. The support of celebrities is as disgusting as the habit. How can you peddle a product that hooks and kills so many (unless you work in the fishing industry)?

Second-hand Smoke

Despite enormous amounts of scientific proof to the contrary, many cling to the mistaken notion that second-hand smoke (also called passive smoke) is harmless. They usually have a financial interest in keeping the addicted puffing.

There is nothing passive about environmental smoke. Even short-term exposure to it has adverse cardiac effects. If you can smell it, it can harm you. Anyone with heart disease should avoid smoke-filled rooms. Long-term exposure accounts for thousands of deaths per year from heart disease and lung cancer. There are two types of second-hand smoke, **mainstream smoke** (15% of the total smoke), which is exhaled by the culprit, and **sidestream smoke** (the remaining 85%), which comes from the end of the cigarette between puffs. Sidestream smoke is more dangerous since the particles released are smaller and more likely to become trapped in the lungs. Therefore, if a smoker won't butt out, ask them to blow the smoke directly in your face to spare you exposure from the more dangerous sidestream smoke.

Children

Statistics won't go away. Smoking is associated with a greater risk of miscarriages, stillbirths, smaller babies, early childhood death (including sudden infant death syndrome), and more childhood lung problems. Smoking during and after pregnancy impairs a child's proper lung development. Children in smoke-filled homes are nearly 50% more likely to develop pneumonia and asthma and 20% more likely to develop ear infections than children in smoke-free homes. **Allowing children to inhale second-hand smoke by lighting up in the home or smoking during pregnancy is child abuse.**

Smoking interferes with fertility and lowers the age of menopause. That pregnant women continue to smoke is a testimony to the strength of the addiction. Because I don't smoke, I can never understand its grip, but how a pregnant woman can continue to puff away when she knows the effects on her baby amazes me (did somebody say denial?). In one study, more than a third of the pregnant women who claimed to have quit were discovered to have lied when their urine was tested for evidence of smoking.

Heart & Stroke

With all of these sobering facts, it almost seems superfluous to discuss the cardiovascular effects of smoking. Smoking increases the chances of developing a **stroke**. The effect of a stroke is analogous to that of a heart attack. In a heart attack, blood flow is cut off to a portion of the heart when the vessel is blocked. In a stroke, part of the brain loses its blood supply. The area of the brain affected will determine the effect. Patients may be unable to walk due to paralysis of one side of the body, or they may be rendered speechless. Smokers who have a stroke tend to be about 10 years younger than nonsmokers who suffer a stroke. Seeing an unresponsive bedridden stroke patient lying in diapers and being fed pablum should serve as another impetus to quit.

Smoking is responsible for over 70% of cases of **peripheral vascular disease**, or PVD. PVD is the narrowing of the blood vessels of the limbs, usually the legs, which makes walking painful and may lead to amputation. What about heart disease? The chance of developing coronary artery disease is quadrupled by cigarettes and is dose-dependent. The more you smoke, the more likely you will develop heart problems. Smokers with coronary disease are three times more likely to die than nonsmokers with it. Living with a smoker can also be dangerous to your health. Nonsmoking men whose wives smoke have twice the cardiac death rates as husbands of nonsmokers.

Quitting —
It's (Almost) Never Too Late

The benefits of quitting cigarettes are surprising. The mortality rate from smoking-related coronary artery disease drops by 50% within one year. After 10 years of abstinence, it approaches the risk of lifelong nonsmokers. Within three years of becoming smoke-free (before age 55, though), the chance of having a heart attack decreases to the same level as that of nonsmokers. The risk of lung cancer, stroke, and emphysema decrease more slowly. By about 15 years after quitting, the cancer risk approaches (though never equals) that of nonsmokers. Of course the road is paved with some discarded cigarette butts. Because nicotine suppresses **leptin**, a hormone responsible for appetite, people who quit gain an average of 10 pounds, with men adding slightly more weight. This occurs in about 80% of quitters, and the thinner you are, the more weight you are likely to gain.

An Addiction

Smoking is a psychologically and physically addictive habit involving tolerance and dependency. **A pack-a-day smoker takes over 80,000 hits of nicotine a year.** A hit takes under 10 seconds to reach the pleasure centres of the brain. A pack-a-day smoker chokes on nearly 350,000 cigarettes in 40 years, administering 3–4 million hits of nicotine during that time.

Smoking is a complex interplay of personal, social, and physical dependency. Despite the protests of those who make a living from it, nicotine is an extremely addictive drug. Addiction represents a loss of control over smoking behaviour. Choosing to smoke may not be as simple as choosing an item from a menu, but it is still a choice. Though five out of six people wish they could quit, they puff because they like to. It's no different than unprotected sex, except there's more phlegm (with smoking). There are a number of excellent programs to assist a smoker on the road to abstention. The decision to pursue such programs is the hardest part. The choice will always be with the individual.

Nicotine causes tolerance, meaning more and more is required to achieve the same effects. As any smoker will attest, withdrawal involves powerful symptoms and intense cravings for tobacco. It may be associated with depression, insomnia, irritability, anxiety, and difficulty concentrating. These symptoms can interfere with relationships at home and at work. Symptoms of withdrawal begin within hours of the last cigarette. They usually peak in a few days and may last months. The greatest risk of relapse is during the first two weeks after quitting, when withdrawal symptoms are most severe. Smoking also causes psychological dependency, providing relaxation during periods of stress and a jump start during less energetic times. Nicotine improves reaction time, short-term memory, and alertness, but so does an extra hour of sleep. Any attempt to quit must address both physical and psychological dependence.

How to Quit

Most people fail one or two serious attempts at quitting smoking before succeeding. A history of a previously failed try is important because it indicates ongoing motivation to butt out. People who successfully quit smoking tend to go through five stages: **pre-contemplation** ("One of these days I am going to quit this stinking habit"), **contemplation** ("I am going to quit this stinking habit"), **preparation** ("I better go see my doctor so I can figure out how to quit this stinking habit"), **action** ("Hi, Doc"), and **abstinence** ("No, I can't bum you a smoke — I quit"). The most important part of any program aimed at encouraging smoking cessation is motivation. The addicted smoker must be motivated to quit before starting the program.

What are the rates of success? About one third of smokers try to quit each year. Under 10% of those who quit for one day remain cigarette-free after one year. The following quitting techniques are available:

1. Advice and encouragement
2. Cognitive-behaviour therapy

3. Abrupt cessation (cold turkey)
4. Nicotine replacement therapy, or NRT
   (the gum, the patches, and the inhaler)
5. Medication
6. Acupuncture
7. Gradual cessation
8. Hypnosis

An important reason people find it so difficult to quit relates to **conditioning**. The cigarette becomes associated with social events, a glass of alcohol, or a cup of coffee. Like Pavlov's dog, which salivated in response to the sound of a bell instead of the sight of food, smokers feel an urge to light up just by being in certain social situations. Failure to address conditioning is a common cause of relapse among initially successful quitters. They haven't had a cigarette in months, but when they step inside a bar they can't fight the urge to light up.

Slick advertising associates smoking with beauty, slimness, adventure, and success. This type of conditioning draws in legions of new smokers and makes it tougher for them to quit. It should be associated with wrinkles, bad breath, missing teeth, and death, but such honesty wouldn't meet the bottom line.

In an analysis of 52 separate studies in which smokers were given **advice** and **encouragement**, about 98% relapsed by one year, and encouragement (e.g., "Light that cigarette and I'll rip out your larynx!") added nothing to advice alone. In a further 30 trials involving nonspecific behaviour modification, including consultations with psychiatrists, again only 2% quit. As a testament to the power of nicotine as well as the 4,000 or so other components of cigarettes, the rate at which high risk groups quit is startling. With advice, 8% of pregnant women, 21% of men deemed to be "high risk," and 36% of survivors of heart attacks were cigarette-free at one year. Non-survivors had a 100% quit rate.

Hypnosis has shown only very modest results when used alone. Multiple sessions of hypnosis, when used as an adjunct to more proven techniques, may enhance the benefits of other more serious forms of therapy. **Acupuncture** and the **gradual cessation** method have also been commercially touted as effective strategies. These have been rigorously and scientifically assessed in at least eight trials each. Neither method had any effect compared to no strategy at all. There will always be those who swear by these techniques, but at present there is no proof that they work. But a drowning man will grab the point of a sword, so I don't expect them to become any less popular. The message is that very few people are able to quit and simple advice or an acupuncture or hypnosis session is hopelessly inadequate. The most a physician can do is provide information which will hopefully lead to the pursuit of a more effective strategy for quitting.

An initial step for those who wish to quit is to simply pick a "quit date." This is effective in up to 20% of motivated individuals. Others need formal behaviour therapy in smoking cessation clinics. No one therapy can be described as the most successful. One of the more interesting behaviour therapies is satiation, a form of **aversion therapy**. The smoker is supposed to take a puff every six seconds. This is like forcing someone with a sweet tooth to polish off a box of chocolates in two minutes (I could do that, if they were low fat). Another behavioural therapy is **self-monitoring**, which is a personal smoking diary. There are also various voluntary agencies, community programs, videos, and pamphlets available to assist the smoker in quitting.

Nicotine Replacement

Many years ago, the idea of **nicotine replacement** was hatched. Because nicotine is responsible for the addiction, supplying it in another form without the cancer-causing agents (carcinogens) of tobacco sounded promising. This concept fulfilled its expectations, and NRT (**nicotine replacement therapy**) is a mainstay of treatment. Though NRT sounds simple, there are a number of pitfalls. The amount of nicotine prescribed (in a patch, gum, or spray) is determined by the degree of dependence. A simple method to assess this is the Fagerstrom test for nicotine dependence (table 32). If a patient scores more than 6, there is significant dependence and a higher likelihood of severe withdrawal symptoms. Therefore a higher dose of NRT will likely be required.

NRT provides a slow and constant release of nicotine into the blood. This contrasts with the rapid short bursts of nicotine that cigarettes provide. Used properly, NRT raises blood nicotine levels to about one half of those reached with cigarettes. NRT reduces the physical withdrawal symptoms of quitting. Among those smokers simply offered the therapy, only 4% quit permanently. Twice as good as advice alone but still abysmal. Therefore NRT is of minimal use by itself. NRT should be used as a companion to a formal smoking cessation program and physician support. When NRT, physician advice, and formal behaviour modification are undertaken together, the quit rate reaches a respectable 30%. Nicotine replacement comes in two main forms: skin patches and gum. Patches are marginally more successful than gum.

Gum & Patches: A Users' Guide

Gum comes in two strengths, 2 mg and 4 mg. It must be chewed thoroughly to maximize nicotine absorption. The amount of chewing required is a real mouth workout and can fatigue the jaw, though you won't get bulging jaw muscles.

1. One piece of 2 mg gum should be chewed for 30–45 minutes for every two cigarettes smoked. If more than 20 cigarettes are smoked per day, or the score on

the Fagerstrom test is high, then benefit can only be expected with 4 mg pieces chewed for every three to four cigarettes smoked.

2. A regular chewing schedule is important to ensure maximum benefit. The dose of gum and frequency of chewing can be weaned after six weeks.

3. Some people develop a dependence on the gum. Five percent of all users and 15% of those who successfully quit smoking are still chewing nicotine gum after a year.

Patches are nicotine delivery systems in which the nicotine is absorbed through the skin. Various formulations exist, including Nicoderm, Habitrol, Nicotrol, and Prostep.

1. A patch is applied once per day to non-hairy and dry skin (not non-dry hairy skin). The site should be changed daily and the same site should not be used for five days.

2. Hands should be washed after the application as nicotine can be irritating to the eyes and mouth (yours and your loved ones').

3. Nicoderm is a 10-week system in which a 21 mg patch is used daily for six weeks, then a 14 mg patch for two weeks, and a 7 mg patch for the remaining two weeks.

4. Habitrol patches come in the same strengths, though the system is prescribed over four weeks.

5. For those who smoke more than 10 cigarettes per day, the highest dosage should be used. If less than 10 are smoked per day, the middle dose is used, and if less than five cigarettes are smoked per day, withdrawal symptoms are unlikely and the patch is generally not beneficial.

Side effects of gum and patches may include insomnia, abnormal dreams, anxiety, nausea, flu-like symptoms, diarrhea, and heartburn. With all forms of NRT, it is dangerous to continue smoking because nicotine toxicity may occur, manifested by nausea, lightheadedness, and seizures. Simply filling out a prescription without other supports in place often results in failure. A quit date should be set and adhered to. NRT reduces physical symptoms of nicotine withdrawal along the road to abstinence, and should not be used in isolation.

FAGERSTROM TEST FOR NICOTINE ADDICTION

Questions and Answers   *Score (out of 10)**

1. How soon after you wake up do you smoke your first cigarette?
    — less than 5 minutes 3
    — 6–30 minutes 2
    — 31–60 minutes 1
    — more than 60 minutes 0
2. Is it difficult for you to refrain from smoking in places where it is forbidden (e.g., at the movies)?
    — yes 1
    — no 0
3. Which cigarette would you hate to give up most?
    — first in the morning 1
    — any other 0
4. How many cigarettes per day do you smoke?
    — more than 31 3
    — 21–30 2
    — 11–20 1
    — less than 10 0
5. Do you smoke more in the first hours after awakening than the rest of the day?
    — yes 1
    — no 0
6. Do you smoke even when you are so sick you have to remain in bed most of the day?
    — yes 1
    — no 0

*scores over 6 indicate significant nicotine addiction and scores under 6 may still reflect addiction.

In terms of safety, there is no evidence that using the gum or patch will increase the likelihood of having a heart attack. In a study of patients with a history of stable angina (meaning predictable symptoms), no harm resulted from these medications. These drugs are classified as unsafe for pregnant women due to the level of nicotine released, though it is less than one half the level reached with smoking actual cigarettes.

Nicotine Inhalers

Other nicotine delivery systems are being tested, and these include nasal sprays, lozenges, and vapor inhalers. Nicotine inhalers have been approved for prescription use. They are designed like cigars and cigarettes, and provide a "hit" of nicotine with each inhalation. Smoking the inhaler, without the rest of the toxins released from tobacco, mimics the oral pleasure of the habit. These devices are twice as effective as placebo inhalers in helping smokers kick the habit.

Medication

Recent preliminary data shows that an antidepressant medication called **bupoprion** is quite effective in getting smokers to quit. It is now being compared with more conventional nicotine replacement therapy.

Conclusion

Aside from financial profit, cigarettes provide no benefit. The leading tobacco manufacturers in North America are Phillip Morris and RJR Nabisco. In 1992, the Phillip Morris Company was the number-one profit-generating business in the United States in 1992 with sales of $50 billion and profits of $4.9 billion. That's a heck of a corporate bonus to management. Cash is the bottom line. It is a sobering realization that the money generated by the tobacco industry is so vast and lines so many pockets that the only hope of restricting its use is through the court system (where lawyers will have their pockets lined instead).

Quitting is possible. Millions do it every year, though many more die an early, addicted death. I hope this chapter assists you in your journey to join the legions of former smokers who have successfully broken the stranglehold of tobacco.

POINTS TO REMEMBER

- **Tobacco (cigarettes, cigars, and pipes) causes more diseases than there are pages in this book. Though it is true that some smokers live to a ripe old age, some passengers survive plane crashes, too.**

- **Second-hand smoke may be mainstream or sidestream and is responsible for tens of thousands of deaths from cancer and heart disease.**

- **Quitting will quickly reduce the risk of cancer and heart disease, but due to physical and psychological addiction and withdrawal symptoms, very few people are successful without help.**

- **Conditioning is the association of the bad habit with other situations, like coffee, sex, or alcohol. It has to be addressed by the successful quitter.**

- **Nicotine replacement therapy (gum, patches, inhaler) has a low success rate by itself. Behaviour modification with physician support should be undertaken simultaneously.**

15

REVERSING HEART DISEASE

It is only fitting that the final chapter revolves around the mysterious concept of regression. I am not referring to past life regression, but rather the regression of coronary artery disease. Think of it as a means to avoid "past lives" with delay tactics.

This book explains how to control your cardiac risk factors, but can you reverse the damage that has already been done? It is only natural that once diagnosed with coronary artery disease, many patients want to know if the narrowings are reversible. The short answer is yes. Regrettably, this cannot be accomplished with simplistic naturopathic or herbal deceptions. The goal can be achieved only through the aggressive application of scientifically validated lifestyle changes as detailed throughout this book.

There are countless studies which have investigated the regression of coronary disease. The strongest are those which looked at coronary arteries with angiograms before and after a drug or dietary intervention. Angiograms are the most direct way to assess the effectiveness of a treatment. In a coronary angiogram, pictures are taken of the blood vessels. Patients are then treated (perhaps with a lipid-lowering drug), and further pictures are taken after a predetermined period of time.

There have been a number of important trials in the field of regression. The most noteworthy are MARS, REGRESS, FATS, SCRIP, POSCH, MAAS, CCAIT, STARS, CLAS, NHLBI type II, UC-SCOR, Lifestyle Heart Trial, and Heidelberg. The acronyms for these trials are often feeble attempts to create a medical catchword to immortalize a study. For example, if a trial looked at the Effect of **D**iet on **C**oronary **A**rtery **D**isease **R**egression, you could call it EDCADR. Not too catchy. But what if you called it "**F**ollowing **A**therosclerosis **R**egression **T**rial?" A lot catchier. What I would like to do now is review each of these trials in minute detail in ancient Greek, including the favourite colours and heights of the lead investigators. Maybe not.

Let's jump right to the conclusions instead. Taken together, these studies have proven that lowering cholesterol not only increases the chances of halting progression of atherosclerosis, but also increases the chances of reversing it. **More specifically, lipid-lowering drugs, used alone or in combination with dietary therapy, lower blood cholesterol levels and increase the likelihood of reversing coronary disease.** Regular exercise is also useful in turning back the clock.

Unfortunately, regression is not guaranteed by lowering lipids. Though following the advice contained in this book will tremendously increase your chances of living your life free of serious heart disease, the solution to the problem is not that simple. When an appendix is inflamed, removing it is curative. When coronary artery disease develops, simply removing the fat with a lipidectomy is not (yet) possible.

Conclusion

Identifying just who will benefit most from drugs and lifestyle changes is beyond physicians at this time. The more vigilant you are in dealing with your risks, the more likely you will prevent CAD, halt its progression or reverse it. Simply focussing on a single risk such as lipids is inadequate. You must think about your **global risk** to develop a coherent strategy to reduce your odds of developing coronary disease.

Such a strategy includes the following considerations:

1) Obtain your lipid profile.
2) Check your blood pressure.
3) Eat intelligently.
4) Exercise safely and regularly.
5) Quit smoking.
6) Consider hormone replacement therapy (women only).
7) Drink a daily glass of alcohol.

To some physicians, the study of medicine is an interest; to others, it is a passion. The same categories apply to the patients I deal with daily. Many are passionate about taking control of their disease. They are willing to do what must be done to alter their risk. The premise of this book is simple. Risk-factor modification is an integral part of the therapeutic approach. It can be accomplished easily. Once your decision is made, all you need is determination and this book. I sincerely hope your interest has been transformed into a passion.

From alcohol to vitamins, you have read about the various ways to modify your cardiac risk factors. I encourage you to read this book over and over again to solidify these concepts. I promise you that your chances of developing heart disease are lower now than they were before you began this journey. The more changes you implement, the healthier you will be. Take control!

GLOSSARY

angina — Pain secondary to reduced blood flow through the heart's arteries. It is not necessarily chest pain but rather may be felt in various locations, including the arm, throat, or back. Its most central definition is that it is cardiac in origin.

angioplasty — Angio means blood vessel and plasty means to fix. A small balloon is dilated over a narrowing in an artery to compress the narrowing and allow more blood to flow. Though angioplasty is commonly performed on the coronary arteries, various other arteries in the body are amenable to this procedure.

antioxidants — Compounds which act as scavengers within cells. They pick up and neutralize nasty by-products of normal metabolism. Some *may* help protect us from developing heart disease.

artery — Takes blood full of oxygen from the heart to the brain and body.

asystole — No heartbeat at all. Unconsciousness would ensue in 10 seconds.

atherosclerosis — Narrowings or complete blockages in arteries due to a buildup of fat in the walls.

atrium — One of two small chambers in the heart which accept blood from the body (right atrium) and the lungs (left atrium) and then propels it to the major chambers of the heart, the ventricles.

bradycardia — A very slow heartbeat, defined as less than 60 beats per minute. Many people normally are "bradycardic."

cardiac — Relating to the heart.

cardiovascular — A general term referring to the blood vessels in the body and the heart.

CHF — Congestive heart failure, characterized by an inability of the heart to pump blood throughout the body, often because it is weakened by heart attacks.

cholesterol — A type of fat, it is only found in foods of animal origin. Blood levels are directly correlated with coronary artery disease.

circumflex artery — One of the main blood vessels supplying the heart.

cigarette — Money to some, death to others.

CK (**creatinine kinase**) — An enzyme which exists in various cells of the body in different forms. The heart has a unique form which is released into the blood when the heart cells die, as in a heart attack. Detection of CK thus becomes a useful way to diagnose heart attacks.

coronary arteries — The blood vessels which supply blood (i.e., nourishment) to the heart muscle.

diabetes — A disease characterized by high blood sugar levels.

diastolic — A time period when the heart is relaxing and blood is pouring into it.

HDL — Stands for high density lipoprotein and is one of the good carriers of various fats within the bloodstream.

heart rate — The number of heartbeats in a minute.

hydrogenated vegetable oils — Sounds healthy but it is exactly the opposite. These are vegetable oils which have been chemically modified by hydrogenation, making them saturated and thus atherogenic.

hypertension — High blood pressure.

LDL — Stands for low density lipoprotein and is one of the bad carriers of various fats in the bloodstream.

left anterior descending artery (LAD) — One of the major blood vessels supplying the heart.

left main artery — A short segment of artery which gives rise to all the blood supply of the left side of the heart (the left anterior descending and circumflex arteries).

lipid — Fat.

lipoprotein — A protein which carries cholesterol and triglycerides through the bloodstream to various sites in the body, like a convoy of transport trucks carting produce between cities.

monounsaturated fats — Dietary fats which may have a role in lowering blood cholesterol levels. They have a different chemical structure than polyunsaturated and saturated fats.

myocardial infarction — Heart attack.

myocardium — Fancy word for the actual heart muscle. Bicep is the muscle of the arm and myocardium is the muscle of the heart.

nitroglycerin — A drug used to dilate the blood vessels of the heart so that more blood can pass through.

plaque — A fatty deposit which narrows blood vessels.

polyunsaturated fats — These are called essential dietary fats because the body cannot manufacture them. They include omega-3 and omega-6. Their intake has been linked to a lower incidence of coronary disease.

right coronary artery (RCA) — One of the major blood vessels supplying the heart.

saturated fats — These dietary fats can be thought of as "hidden" fats. They raise blood cholesterol and are hidden in many processed foods. They should be avoided.

systolic — A time period when the heart is contracting and thus pushing out blood.

tachycardia — A fast heartbeat, usually defined as more than 100 beats per minute.

transfatty acids — Another byproduct of chemical processing, these fats raise blood cholesterol levels and are very dangerous. There is no legislation requiring they be listed on packages.

triglyceride — One form of lipids and found in most foods.

ventricle — One of two main pumping chambers of the heart. The right ventricle pumps blood to the heart, and the left to the body.

ventricular tachycardia — An extremely fast and dangerous heart rhythm which is initiated in the main pumping chamber of the heart, the ventricle, instead of the normal place, the atrium. It is frequently 150–250 beats a minute.

vein — Takes blood from which much of the oxygen has been removed, and returns the blood back to the heart, which in turn sends the blood to the lungs for an oxygen refill.

VLDL — Stands for very low density lipoprotein.